Should I FIRE My Doctor?

Eleven Essential Elements to
Health and Happiness

Patricia J Sulak MD

Founder, Living WELL Aware™

and a

Physician, Researcher, Professor, and Patient

Should I FIRE My Doctor?
Eleven Essential Elements to Health and Happiness

Founder, Living WELL Aware™
and a Physician, Researcher, Professor, and Patient

Published by Next Century Publishing
www.NextCenturyPublishing.com

ISBN: 978-162-9030562

Printed in the United States of America

Contact the author at: www.livingwellaware.com

Endorsements

This book is essential reading for anyone who wishes to take the quality of their life to an even higher level. Since I am married to the author, I know more than anyone else about the tremendous passion and enthusiasm Patsy brings to the subject of wellness! *Should I Fire My Doctor?* encapsulates the principles by which we live each day, and I am now happier and more energetic than I've ever been. Join me on the exciting journey of creating the very best possible version of yourself. You'll be glad you did.

—Jeffrey A. Waxman, MD

Should I Fire My Doctor? is a great read. Dr Sulak highlights how our culture has negatively impacted our health, offers proven healthier choices, and highlights her own life changes. While her motivational and entertaining Living WELL Aware conference should be on everyone's bucket list, her book is definitely a stand-alone path to greater health and happiness.

Bethany Black MD, Pediatrician

I have worked with thousands of leaders all over the world as an executive coach and wish I would have had this book for all of them to read. It provides the missing answers as to how you can achieve real life balance and have the energy you need to accomplish your goals. I also was fortunate enough to attend a Living Well Aware workshop with Dr Sulak and the only thing better than studying her book was a healthy dose of her energy and the wisdom of the plan she presented. This is now on the required reading list for all of my clients.

—Bill Moyer, Co-Founder and CEO
SOS Leadership Institute, LLC

I am very excited about Dr. Sulak's book, *Should I Fire My Doctor?* Dr. Sulak is one of the leading physicians in the United States and this book provides the scientifically proven medical and psychological principles of self-care as presented in her Living Well Aware courses. Written in a very practical manner, this information packed guide will be of tremendous help to the millions of people who are interested in learning how to achieve their optimal health. Read this book and you will have the basis for better health and more happiness!

—Gary Elkins, Ph.D., ABPP, ABPH
Professor, Department of Psychology and Neuroscience
Director, Clinical Psychology Program
Director, Mind-Body Medicine Research Laboratory
Baylor University
Waco, Texas
Author of *Relief From Hot Flashes: The Natural, Drug-Free Program to Reduce Hot Flashes, Improve Sleep, and Ease Stress*

Acknowledgements

This book became a reality because of the loving encouragement of my amazing husband of 33 years, Dr. Jeffrey Waxman. Our journey to optimal health and happiness led to the creation of our Living WELL Aware conferences and *Should I Fire My Doctor?* book. We continue to faithfully travel this road together.

Thanks also to our son, Bart Waxman, for his advice and legal assistance in the creation of Living WELL Aware, and to our son, Gabe Waxman, who created the logo and marketing materials to get the program going. It has truly been a family project.

Dedication

This book is dedicated to healthcare professionals who have devoted their lives to helping others. Often faced with declining reimbursement, time constraints and mounting administrative responsibilities, they continue to tirelessly care for a population that is becoming progressively unhealthy and unhappy. It is my hope this book will be a catalyst for these dedicated professionals—both personally and professionally—to motivate their patients and themselves towards the goal of Living WELL Aware.

Should I Fire My Doctor? is also dedicated to those who strive to be living examples of the health and happiness that is possible by taking ownership of all aspects of our lives. Continuing the journey of Living WELL Aware will move us closer to reaching the potential we are all capable of being.

Foreword

As with most people, my life became way too busy. Then one day, I realized I couldn't walk up a set of stairs without becoming winded. I realized I had begun planning my days to avoid stairs and even walking. My weight and general health decline had suddenly become the deciding factor for how I existed each day. That was it! I began the search for answers to help me make life-saving changes.

I found a new doctor, got a physical, and worked with her to reach specific goals on blood pressure and weight. I also attended a wellness seminar lead by Dr. Patsy Sulak.

I did not know what to expect. But during the course of the day Patsy taught me that I *can* control my destiny, and it's not too late for me to make changes. She shared her personal journey and search for health and a well-rounded life, and invited every participant to find healthcare professionals who would be honest and straightforward about what it would take for each of us to reach specific goals, and achieve results in fitness, wellness and emotional well-being. That day I learned that I am my most important healthcare provider, and my job was to move *every day for the rest of my life for at least an hour, seek support and reinforcement, and set specific but realistic goals for my lifestyle.*

Armed with new tennis shoes and a new attitude, I began walking. My legs became stronger, as did my resolve to become healthier in every way with every step.

Then the unthinkable happened shortly after attending this seminar. My husband of over 20 years died from an apparent heart attack. He was overweight, in poor physical condition, and suffered from high blood pressure. While consumed with grief, I continued to walk, and walk some more, and focused on what I had learned in Patsy's one-day seminar. The walking was nurturing—an unintended effect on my emotional wellness and ability to handle this change and loss of a loved one—and offered me time to reflect on changes my husband could have made, and changes I could make moving forward.

I was so inspired and determined by Patsy and my friends that I have now walked in my first 5K, lowered my blood pressure, and lost 35 pounds! My leg strength has improved to the point that I don't even think about taking a flight of stairs.

Thank you Patsy for sharing your wisdom and personal stories, and for teaching others that it is never too late, if you are willing to change!

I am armed with information and inspiration from the Living WELL Aware conference, from this book, and from great doctors who provide support on this new journey. While I cannot change things for my husband, I know that, with determination and focus, I am inspired to help myself and others live a healthier lifestyle with every step by Living WELL Aware.

—Mary Black Pearson, J.D.

Table of Contents

Introduction

Should you fire your doctor or primary care provider? This is a legitimate question. Is your doctor (MD, DO), nurse practitioner (NP), or physician assistant (PA) maximizing your health or doing no more than simply diagnosing and treating disease? As a practicing physician, researcher, medical school professor, and patient, I find health a major focus of my life—professionally and personally. After thirty years of clinical practice, I am seeing a different patient population now than I did in my earlier years of practice. And it's not good.

Despite our conveniences at home and at work, despite countless life-saving advances in medicine, our waiting rooms are filled with patients who are not healthy, not happy, and even depressed. They often have self-inflicted medical conditions including obesity, diabetes, and numerous other risk factors for disease and disability. Many are complicating their lives and harming their well-being with numerous unhealthy behaviors including a sedentary lifestyle, dietary indiscretion, tobacco use, drug abuse, and self-induced stress often leading to anxiety and depression.

These health risk behaviors can lead to cardiovascular disease (CVD), the #1 killer of Americans. Here are some facts released by the Centers for Disease Control and Prevention (CDC) and other medical institutions that should alarm all of us:

- The majority of deaths (over 70 percent) in adolescents and young adults ages 10-24 are due to accidents, murder and suicide.
- The death rates for ages 25-34 *increased* in 2011.
- The suicide rate for ages 35-64 *increased* 30 percent over the last few years.
- In 2013, the CDC announced that there is a "Painkiller Epidemic Among Women" with almost one million emergency department visits by women for drug misuse and abuse.
- There are now more deaths in the U.S. from drug overdoses than from motor vehicle accidents.
- Obesity is an epidemic with two-thirds of the U.S. population overweight and half of those obese, increasing risks for multiple health problems including diabetes, heart attacks, strokes, degenerative joint disease, and even some cancers.

I could go on and on with more startling medical facts that are a wake-up call to the current state of health in the United States and other industrialized countries. If the healthcare profession is responsible for the health of our country, it looks like we are flunking. The truth is healthcare professionals are often not good examples of what constitutes a healthy lifestyle. The majority of people in the healthcare industry do not eat a healthy diet or follow the recommendations for physical activity. Most would not call their lives "stress free." The bottom line: *Is the healthcare profession responsible for our health and happiness?*

Where is the problem? What is the answer to this current health decline? The answer is *not* with our healthcare providers. As a busy physician, I can tell you we simply do not have the time during a clinic appointment to give you all the necessary up-to-date medical guidelines and wellness information to maximize your physical and emotional health. We definitely do not have adequate time to assist you in ways to implement the information or to inspire you to make the necessary changes.

With time restraints allotted to each patient, we must focus on diagnosis and treatment of disease, not prevention of disease. "Take this medicine." "Schedule this surgery." It only takes a few seconds to write a prescription for a drug to lower your cholesterol, blood pressure, or glucose level or treat your mood disorder or pain. Most surgical procedures can be done through small incisions in a matter of minutes.

However, it takes many hours to give you all the guidelines and implementation strategies to lead a healthy life to prevent health disorders in the first place. Time doesn't allow us to discuss healthy food consumption recommendations, exercise fitness guidelines, stress reduction techniques, and available tobacco, alcohol, and other addictive cessation programs. In fact, with today's electronic health record system, healthcare providers have to allot more time inputting orders and information into a database, rather than spending one-on-one time with their patients.

The amount of time and reimbursement a provider spends with each patient has remained the same, or has been decreased, while the amount of administrative work they must do has increased in most practices.

So, what is the answer? As consumers of this industry we call the medical field, we need to become educated in health and wellness. What **is** healthy? What **is not** healthy? And, most important: what can we do about it?

Wellness is a multi-billion-dollar industry. Billions of dollars are spent annually on herbs, supplements, vitamins, minerals, and other "health" products, all with convincing ads telling us they can cure anything and everything that ails us with no harmful effects.

Unfortunately, many of these health claims are not backed by published data in respected medical journals. In addition, billions more are spent on prescription medications and surgical procedures, many of which could have been avoided or minimized with a healthy lifestyle. By no means am I discounting the importance of supplements, medications, and surgical procedures. I have found them necessary and beneficial during my own life. I am saying they should *not* be a replacement for Living WELL Aware.

If we want optimal health, we must establish a partnership with a healthcare provider who is vested in assisting us to the level of health we desire. This is what I refer to as, "Partnering With Your Provider." We need to know what has been proven to decrease our likelihood of disease, depression, disability, and death. We also need to know how to implement guidelines and how our healthcare provider and others can assist and inspire us.

That is the purpose of this book's discussion of Eleven Essential Elements of Health and Happiness. As is often said, "Knowledge is Power." Knowing the most current, factual, published medical **Information** is the first step to getting on the path of leading a healthier and happier life. But to progress down the path, we need proven **Implementation** options to apply the information we have learned. And, to stay on the path, we need continual **Inspiration**.

I have no "health" products to sell you. My goal is that by Living WELL Aware, we will reduce the number of over-the-counter supplements, prescription medications, healthcare office visits, and surgical procedures we all need during our lifetime. With the current constraints on healthcare access in this country due to our current multi-trillion dollar deficit, it behooves all of us to do everything we can to implement scientifically proven strategies to decrease our need for the services of the healthcare industry.

I am a medical school professor, published researcher, national medical speaker, practicing physician, wife of a practicing physician, mother, and a patient. I have used all of these roles to put together a truly unique wellness conference entitled Living WELL Aware: Habits That Lead to Health and Happiness. This book summarizes the information given to attendees in this one-day conference.

As a medical school professor and researcher, I am dedicated to finding the very best and latest medical information on the components of scientifically proven healthy living. As a practicing physician and teacher, I strive to convey this information to patients and healthcare professionals in an entertaining, inspiring fashion. As a patient whose goal is to achieve optimal physical, emotional, and spiritual health, I search for the many ways to implement the vast information available into our daily lives, no matter where we are starting or where we want to see ourselves individually.

This book is for everyone: men and women, thin and obese, happy and depressed, athletic and out of shape, health aware and health unaware. No matter where we are right now, we can all get to a greater level of health and happiness. That is the ultimate goal of this book: one step at a time, one person at a time, turning the current culture of convenience and harm to a culture of accountability and health. We can do it, but only if we are Living WELL Aware and have the very best in wellness information, implementation, and inspiration to get us there. Only then will you be able to find a healthcare professional to Partner with Your Provider to maximize your health.

Let's work with healthcare professionals who are invested in their own health and ours, not only diagnosing and treating disease but actively working to prevent disease. Welcome to Living WELL Aware.

CAUTIONARY WORDS!

Before we begin laying out the Living WELL Aware "Eleven Essential Elements to Health and Happiness," a few cautionary words are in order. They are not really "disclaimers" but rather important points that allow readers to discern how to apply the information to their own lives.

1) One size does not fit all

You might ask how I came up with these eleven elements to consider incorporating into one's life. As a physician, teacher, researcher, and importantly, a patient who is pursuing the best in living life to its fullest, I work on these elements in my own life.

I have not only searched the world's literature on what is healthy, but am successfully applying these concepts to my life with dramatic results. Many attendees of my Living WELL Aware conferences have also sung the praises of this "Information, Implementation, and Inspiration" with life-changing results.

You may find each and every one helpful. I hope you do—and think you will. But remember, this is *my* list. Add, subtract, and edit as fits *your* unique life. One of the goals of this book is to develop a strong foundation on which you can build. While the recommendations given can be applied to the overwhelming majority, some may not apply to individuals with specific characteristics, health disorders, or personal or religious beliefs. Do not hesitate to consult healthcare professionals and others regarding specific recommendations for your concerns.

2) Stay informed

The information and recommendations discussed are up to date as of the publication date. Some of the information was released only a few months prior to this book's completion.

We are learning new information about what constitutes a healthy and unhealthy lifestyle at an astounding pace. Stay informed and utilize reputable sources.

3) Get clearance

If you are reading this book and have no earthly idea what your health status truly is, remedy that deficit quickly with a checkup from a healthcare provider who is vested in her personal wellness and yours. If you have a muscle and/or joint problem, go for evaluation. This is especially important when beginning a physical fitness program.

If you have breathing difficulties, high blood pressure or other disorders or risk factors for cardiovascular disease that will be discussed here, address them first to make sure you don't kill yourself trying to be healthy! Err on the side of caution when it comes to your health and get clearance.

4) Don't ditch your drugs

This book focuses on disease prevention through lifestyle modifications. While pharmaceutical therapies will not be discussed, their importance in reducing death and disability are well documented and fully supported.

The goal of this book is to hopefully reduce the number of clinic visits, medications, surgeries, and hospitalizations we will need in our lifetime by Living WELL Aware. Do not discontinue a maintenance medication without first discussing it with a respected healthcare professional.

5) Consult "Higher" sources

Spiritual aspects of health and wellness will be discussed with no promotion of any one philosophy or religion. Fortunately, when it comes to aspects of how we should lead our life in pursuing health and happiness, all the major religions and even Greek scholars are largely in agreement. Apply the spiritual aspects of wellness that are discussed based on your own beliefs.

6) Be prepared to be offended

My goal is to offend everyone in some form or fashion by the end of this book! Well, maybe not offend, but at least get under your skin. Believe me, in pursing optimal wellness, I had to question many lifetime habits I needed to alter. I still find it challenging to implement all the aspects of healthy living I will discuss.

If we want to get to the next level of health and happiness, we often have to question something we may have been doing or thinking, possibly for decades. To admit that a long-held action or belief is not serving us well and must be altered or eliminated can first be met with personal resistance.

You'll find this especially true if you and most people you know have bought into it. I invite you to question the suggestions given, study them carefully, and then ask yourself two questions: Is my current belief about this particular aspect of my life serving me well or harming me? Would applying this new information be beneficial to me?

We cannot and will not get better unless we admit something we are doing or believing needs to be changed. That is what Living WELL Aware is all about.

Are Most of Us Healthy
and Happy?

Before we dive into the Eleven Essential Elements to Health and Happiness, let's ask a question. Are most of us healthy and satisfied with our lives? Are we *well*? Let's define *health* and *wellness*.

In 2006, the World Health Organization in "WHO Health Promotion Glossary, New Terms" stated, "*Wellness* is the optimal state of health of individuals and groups, involving not only the realization of the fullest potential of an individual physically, psychologically, socially, spiritually and economically, but also the fulfillment of one's role expectations in the family, community, place of worship, workplace and other settings."

In 1948, the WHO defined *health* as, "A state of complete physical, emotional, and social well-being, and not merely the absence of disease or infirmity." Is anyone out there at the fullest potential of physical, emotional, social, spiritual, and economic health? I'm sure not. Are most of us healthy and happy most of the time?

As a busy physician, my days are filled with patients far from completely content with all aspects of their lives.

These are statements I do **NOT** hear from my patients:

- I'm loving this aging process.
- I hate carbs.
- I'm too happy.
- My sex drive is too high. Please fix it.
- I don't have any trouble controlling my weight.
- I love to exercise.
- I have enough time to get everything done.
- My memory is better than it has ever been.

What I **DO** hear from my patients, over and over:

- I'm tired, lethargic, have no energy.
- I'm stressed, moody, anxious, irritable, and depressed.
- I can't lose weight.
- I can't sleep.
- I have no sex drive.
- I'm in pain.
- I get headaches all the time.
- I'm losing my memory.

OK, you might be one of those people who say, "I don't have any of those complaints. I'm healthy and happy." That's great. But, can you answer **YES** to all of the statements below?

- I'm at my ideal body weight.

- I'm in great physical shape: great endurance, strength, balance, and flexibility.
- I know and am up to date on *all* recommended health screening tests, and they are in the normal range.
- I'm satisfied with my current emotional state. Rarely am I stressed out, moody, anxious, or depressed.
- I harbor anger against no one.
- I have accomplished all of my life goals.
- I am perfect: physically, emotionally, and spiritually!

None of us can answer yes to all of these. None of us are the perfect versions we are capable of being. Therefore, we have room for change and improvement. I find this fact not only challenging but also exciting. We can all get to the next level of health and happiness if we have an accurate road map to get us there, along with a plan to keep us on course.

Let's look at some of the common health disorders:

- Depression/Anxiety/Insomnia
- Headaches/Pain Syndromes
- Diabetes/Obesity/Heart Disease
- High Cholesterol/High Blood Pressure/Stroke
- Acid Reflux/Irritable Bowel/Constipation
- Osteoporosis/Bone Fractures

- Arthritis/Degenerative Joint Disease/Muscle and Joint Disorders
- Alzheimer's Disease/Dementia
- Cancer

There is one thing we can say about all of these health problems: *All* **diseases can be prevented or improved with a healthy lifestyle.** If I am diagnosed with cancer tomorrow, I am going to be better able to deal with that cancer if I am physically, emotionally, and spiritually healthy. My family and friends will also benefit.

It is important for us to know the most common causes of premature death and disability at various ages. We should also know the risk factors and preventative measures for each cause.

Regarding cancer, do you know the most common cause of **cancer deaths** in men? In women? Most people are not aware that the most common cause of cancer deaths in men each year is **lung cancer**, not prostate cancer. The most common cause of cancer deaths in women is also **lung cancer**, not breast cancer. Most lung cancer is preventable if we don't smoke or live/work with smokers.

Most people are aware that the overall **number one cause of death** in men and women is **cardiovascular disease** (heart attacks and strokes). The unfortunate fact is that almost all individuals experiencing a heart attack or stroke had one or more treatable risk factors that could have out-right prevented the event or at least delayed it for many, many years. Wouldn't we all like to live longer and without disability?

I know many of you reading this book are really physically fit. But remember, fitness does not equal health.

A prime example is Jim Fixx, running guru and author of *The Complete Book of Running*. Jim was an inspiration to millions. At the age of 35, he quit smoking, started jogging, and lost fifty pounds. Unfortunately, he did not Partner With His Provider. At the age of 52, despite a high cholesterol level and a strong family history of early heart disease, he declined a cardiac stress test. Unfortunately, he suffered a fatal heart attack while running. His first heart attack was his last and was preventable had he followed the guidelines, which we will discuss in detail. We must all strive to have what I will refer to as, "Normal Numbers Now" when it comes to recommended health-screening tests to dramatically decrease death and disability.

Many of you are up to date on health screening tests and have numbers in the normal range. That's great. But what about other aspects of your life? Are you emotionally where you want to be? Do you feel like there is something missing in your life? How would you rate your significant relationships? Your spirituality? If you are like me, you are eons away from the best you can be.

That is why optimal health is more than physical fitness and more than having perfect health numbers. It is about Living WELL Aware. Let's begin to detail my Eleven Essential Elements of Health and Happiness.

Essential Element #1:

Normal Numbers Now

For achievement of optimal health and maximum longevity, it's critical that we strive for Normal Numbers Now. To what numbers am I referring? While there are many tests that are recommended depending on our age along with personal and family history and gender, all adults should know their own key numbers for:

- Blood pressure
- Cholesterol values
- Fasting blood sugar
- Ideal body weight

Knowing these numbers and getting them in the optimal range can dramatically decrease death and disability. It's also wise to know the normal numbers *and* your own before beginning a physical activity program. Remember Jim Fixx!

Blood Pressure (BP) It's important to diagnose and treat hypertension, the medical term for high blood pressure. Your blood pressure has two numbers: the systolic BP (**SBP**) or top number (think **s**ky) and **d**iastolic BP (**DBP**) or bottom number (think **d**irt) i.e. SBP/DBP. These two values measure the pressure in millimeters of mercury (mm Hg) when your heart is pumping blood through your arteries. Optimally, your SBP should be less than 120 and DBP should be less than 80. A BP of 120/80 or less for each of these numbers is considered normal.

For most of us, lower is better, for example 100 - 110/60 - 70. Can your BP be too low? Only if you are severely dehydrated or hemorrhaging from an accident. A low BP, for example of 90/50, is OK as long as you feel great and do not have a history of heart disease, stroke, anemia, or other illnesses.

High BP should concern all of us. As we age, the majority of us will have elevations in our BP, making yearly evaluation a must to quickly halt further progression and associated problems. Even at BPs of 135/85, over time we are putting ourselves at increased risk of cardiovascular disease (CVD), especially stroke in women.

It is important that we get our BP as close to 120/80 or less by getting to our ideal body weight, exercising, having a low salt diet, and utilizing medications if necessary. Whatever it takes, get your BP as close to normal as possible! By doing so, you may prevent that heart attack or stroke that was otherwise destined to happen down the road if your blood pressure remained elevated and untreated!

Cholesterol Level It is actually a lot more complicated than just knowing that one number. There are several numbers we should know in the group *lipids* or lipid profile. Lipids refer to the fats in our blood, specifically triglycerides and several types of cholesterol. A normal **triglyceride** level is less than 150 milligrams (mg) per deciliter (dL). Triglycerides are often elevated in diabetics and if greatly elevated can cause a severe inflammation of the pancreas (pancreatitis).

The cholesterol in our blood travels primarily on two fat-carrying proteins called lipoproteins: low-density lipoprotein and high-density lipoprotein. Low-density lipoprotein cholesterol (**LDL-C**), found in the plaques in arteries, is often referred to as the bad cholesterol (Lousy or Lethal). The lower the LDL-C the better, with an optimal value of **less than 100 mg/dL.** For individuals at high risk for CVD, it should be less than 70.

High-density lipoprotein cholesterol (**HDL-C**) carries the fat away from the arteries back to the liver, thus giving it the title of good cholesterol (Heavenly or Healthy). **HDL-C** should be **H**igher than **50 mg/dL for women** and **H**igher than **40 mg/dL for men.**

There are other types of cholesterol such as very low-density lipoprotein (VLDL-C), lipoprotein a, and other minor types. These may be important values to know for people with a family history of very early heart attacks or strokes.

Total Cholesterol Your Total Cholesterol is the sum of all the types of cholesterol: Total-C = LDL-C + HDL-C + VLDL-C + lipoprotein a + other minor types of cholesterol. The normal value is said to be less than 200mg/dL but that does not mean all is well if it is below 200. If your heavenly HDL-C is low (which is not good), then your total cholesterol might be less than 200 but that is not a good profile. Or your HDL-C could be really high (which is great) causing your total cholesterol to be greater than 200. Nothing to worry about as long as your LDL-C is normal.

The bottom line: You don't want to know just your Total C. You want to know your LDL-C and HDL-C and you want them in the optimal range if possible.

Fasting Blood Sugar (FBS) or **Fasting Blood Glucose** If the glucose or sugar in our blood is high because our pancreas cannot make enough insulin to get it in a normal range, we have diabetes mellitus (DM). Type I DM often occurs in childhood because of a disorder of the immune system that actually attacks the pancreas causing it not to make enough insulin to keep the blood sugar regulated.

Type 2 DM is often referred to as Adult Onset DM (AODM) and is seen usually in overweight people and certain racial groups. AODM is now also being diagnosed in significantly overweight children because of our current obesity epidemic in all age groups. Our **FBS** should be **less than 100 mg/dL**. If it is between 100 and 126, you have pre-diabetes. If it is over 126 on two separate occasions, you have diabetes. Since diabetes is a major risk factor for CVD, it is important we all know our FBS and get in the normal range.

A FBS only tells us what is going on right at the moment the blood is drawn. If we want to know the average of our blood sugars over the past couple months, we can determine that with a Hemoglobin A 1 C (Hgb A1C). This test gives us the percentage of hemoglobin in the blood that has sugar molecules bound to it. The Hgb A1C should be between 4 and 5.6 percent in people without DM with levels of 6.5 percent or higher indicating DM. Pre-diabetics are between 5.7 and 6.4 percent.

Ideal Body Weight This, the last number that needs to be in the normal range, is the one many people struggle to achieve. Why? It is up to the individual to get it in the normal range. Medications can lower our BP, bad cholesterol, and blood sugar.

Lowering our weight is primarily up to us unless we want to: (1) take medications that usually are ineffective and can have significant side effects and complications, or, (2) have stomach and or bowel surgery which can have serious immediate and lifelong complications.

Our ideal weight is based on our height and calculated from a formula referred to as our body mass index (BMI). It is easy to determine your BMI. Just Google

"BMI calculator" and plug in your weight in pounds and height in inches. Your BMI ideally should be between 18.5 and 25. Greater than 25 and up to 30 is overweight, and a BMI of greater than 30 is considered obese. Later we'll discuss how we can tackle this problem effectively without surgery, medications, injections, or massive exercise.

Do you know your exact numbers? If not, schedule an appointment now to have them calculated. If they are not in the optimal range, get assistance to get them there. We all know people who have had a heart attack or stroke at a young age because they did not understand the importance of Normal Numbers Now. The excuses are numerous:

- "I don't have the time."

Really? Do you have time for a heart attack or stroke?

- "I don't have the money?"

It is inexpensive. There are numerous places to have your tests done for a few bucks—even grocery stores and pharmacies. What is really expensive is being admitted into the hospital!

- "I feel great. My values must be OK."

Wrong! You can have numbers that are off the wall abnormal and feel fine. Once you feel bad, it is often too late. Your first heart attack may be your last!

- "I hate to have my blood drawn, and I hate to go to the doctor."

So do I. That's why I want to know my numbers. If I get them in the normal range, I dramatically decrease my odds of being admitted into the hospital with a heart attack or stroke. That means far *fewer* blood draws and visits!

- "I don't want to take medications for high BP, cholesterol or blood sugar. They have side effects, and they are not natural."

Well, I guess a stroke and even death are "natural." If leading a healthy lifestyle is not adequately correcting your numbers, then medications can help. Work with your healthcare providers to find the treatments that are best for you.

I repeat: Normal Numbers Now! If they are not in the normal range, work with your healthcare provider to get them there. It is an important component of Living WELL Aware!

Essential Element #2:

Critique Caloric Consumption

I, and probably many of you out there, am sick of hearing the word *diet*. It implies drastically decreasing our food intake usually to lose weight while making ourselves miserable in the process. I prefer the term "Critique Caloric Consumption," which implies we simply need to eat healthy and quit consuming crap! We are not only putting an excess number of calories in our body, we are consuming unhealthy food that literally causes death and disability.

Let's discuss today's dual problems: "Excess Intake" and "Unhealthy Intake." We will then discuss the solutions that are easily achievable for anyone who works through all the healthy habits we will discuss.

Excess Intake We put more stuff in our body than most of us can possibly eliminate. Our body is an amazing, efficient machine. It does not want to waste the calories we take in. It was wonderfully programmed thousands of years ago for survival, preparing us for periods of starvation and even famine.

Well, that is not the situation for the overwhelming majority of us who do not live in the Third World. When was the last time we had a famine? Have you gone for days without eating only because of lack of food availability? Our body doesn't know we have an abundance of food. It has maintained its survival capability and stores away any excess calories we take in, preparing us for something that will never happen—starvation!

What is *Excess Intake?* It's not rocket science. Unless we are underweight and need to put on a few pounds, it is simply any calories we take in on a daily basis that we do not burn off. Calories are actually energy units. Calories are consumed and then utilized to run the most amazing machine on the planet—our body. Any calories not consumed in running our body are stored as fat for future use.

Therein lies the problem. It takes no more than a few excess calories each day to cause massive weight gain over time. If you take in only fifty calories each day that your body doesn't burn off, that creates five pounds of weight gain in one year, twenty-five pounds over five years, and fifty pounds over ten years! I have seen this time and time again in my clinical practice.

How did we get into the problem of Excess Intake? Simple—food availability. Food is everywhere! No matter where I go, there is food. I show up to work in the morning and find food in the nurse's station in the hospital. I go to a social function, party or business meeting, and there's food. It seems like someone is always having a birthday, and of course, there's the cake. We celebrate by doing what? Eating and drinking. While millions in the world starve each day, we are literally eating ourselves to death.

In addition to having food everywhere we go, the portion sizes have gone through the roof. Cookies, muffins, hamburgers, spaghetti, pizza, drinks—you name it—can be two or even four times the size they used to be. I'm old enough to remember when a soft drink was six ounces. Then it was 10, 12, 16, 20, 32, and now even 64 ounces!

One cookie at the bakery where I buy groceries could easily feed four people. Unfortunately, people think one cookie is one serving—it isn't! And remember, it only takes 50 extra calories a day to turn into pounds of weight gain each year. That is no more than a few bites of a cookie, pizza, or hamburger or a few swallows of a calorie-laden liquid. That is all it takes.

Unhealthy Intake In addition to having food everywhere we go, in sizes that look like we won't have another chance to eat for days, the calories we take in are often quite unhealthy. We are ruining our food by either adding things to it that make it unhealthy or in the processing of our food. Think about healthy food such as broccoli, corn, tomatoes, chicken, and fish.

We often add cream sauces, turning a healthy food into a high fat, dairy-laden fare with hundreds of additional calories that can increase our weight, cholesterol, blood sugar, and blood pressure. And a salad that is full of lettuce, tomatoes, cucumbers, radishes, and broccoli has gone from being nutrient rich to calorie rich with the addition of a high-fat dairy dressing, croutons, and loads of cheese.

These are extra unhealthy calories that our body does not need, and we won't take time to work off. Much of the food we eat is also processed (i.e., made in a factory) with high-fructose corn syrup added as a sweetener along with a lot of chemicals that you and I have trouble pronouncing.

So what is the result of this Excess Intake and Unhealthy Intake along with a technology laden sedentary culture? It has led to our current obesity epidemic. It happened relatively quickly.

In 1990, every state in the U.S. had an obesity rate of less than 15 percent of its population. Twenty years later, in 2010, *every* state had an obesity rate of over 20 percent with many having obesity rates of 35 percent or greater. Today two-thirds of Americans are overweight, and half of those are obese.

If you are in the normal weight range today, you are the minority.

The medical complications of unhealthy/excess food intake leading to obesity are well substantiated, numerous, and not debatable. The problems of obesity include:

Cardiovascular Risk Factors and Diseases

- Diabetes
- Dyslipidemias (high triglycerides and cholesterol)
- Hypertension (high blood pressure)
- Coronary artery disease (heart attacks, angina)
- Carotid artery disease (transient ischemic attacks, stroke)
- Claudication (pain in the legs due to decreased blood flow)

Pulmonary Diseases

- Obstructive sleep apnea
- Hypoventilation syndrome

Liver/Gall Bladder Diseases

- Fatty-liver disease
- Cirrhosis
- Cholelithiasis (gallstones)

Musculoskeletal Disorders

- Osteoarthritis
- Gout

Gynecologic Disorders

- Abnormal menstruation
- Polycystic ovarian syndrome

- Infertility

Increases in Cancer Risk
- Breast
- Uterus
- Colon
- Esophagus
- Kidney
- Prostate
- Pancreas

Increased surgical complications
- Infection
- Bleeding
- Venous thrombosis (blood clots in veins)
- Cardiovascular complications

I have actually seen the obesity epidemic, along with its multitude of associated health disorders, unfold before me in my practice. I have been working in the same academic healthcare facility in the same town for the past twenty-seven years. Patients I first saw as teenagers are now in their forties, and women who were in their fifties are now in their upper seventies.

No matter what their age when I first saw them, many have slowly but progressively gained weight year after year. They may have started with me weighing 150 pounds but now weigh over 250. How did this happen?

It just slowly crept up on them. As mentioned, it only takes a few extra calories a day (50 calories or even less) for the weight to start piling up in our fat stores.

Patients tell me, "But Dr. Sulak, I don't eat any more than I used to, and I'm still gaining weight." They don't notice the ever-increasing portion sizes at restaurants, fast food establishments, and in processed foods. They don't take into consideration our ever-increasing technology and sedentary social media outlets that decrease our need to move.

Unless you are an alien with some sort of non-human metabolism, we all play by the same rule: energy in/energy out. If you want to gain weight, you are going to have to take in *more* calories than you burn off. If you want to lose weight, you have to take in *fewer* calories than you burn off.

Yes, some people find it easier to lose or gain weight than others. We must each find the level of activity and intake that works for us. After years of trying, I have finally been able to do that. My weight has stayed within three pounds for the last five years with a BMI of 22.

While increasing physical activity will help us lose weight and maintain an ideal BMI, the primary answer to successful weight loss is in the type and amount of food we consume. The overwhelming majority of people just cannot exercise long and hard enough to lose weight solely by using that modality. The effective, expeditious path to overcoming obesity is critiquing caloric consumption and not buying into the cultural norms of unhealthy intake and excess intake. It's a Culture War! We must learn how to eat healthy foods in the amounts we individually need to lose weight, maintain weight, or gain weight.

But what is healthy eating? With so many diets out there promoting weight loss and superior health over all the others, it is difficult for anyone without access to the latest research to know which food plan to undertake for optimal health. The scientific world appears to have a clear answer for us.

The food consumption that has been researched more extensively than any other in very well designed studies is the Mediterranean diet. It is actually not a *diet* as the term usually implies. It is a way of eating. The Mediterranean diet is high in legumes, cereals, fruits, and veggies with fish the primary meat source. The Mediterranean diet is low in dairy products and red meat. There is a high ratio of monounsaturated-fatty acids (like olive oil) compared to saturated-fatty acids (like butter).

While an extensive review of the hundreds of scientific articles published on the benefits of the Mediterranean diet is not the purpose of this book, suffice to say that greater adherence to this food plan has been significantly associated with a reduced risk of death, heart attacks, strokes, cancer, Parkinson's disease, and Alzheimer's disease.

Many articles have been and are continuing to be published in the most reputable journals in the world touting the health benefits of this food consumption. An article published in April 2013, in the *New England Journal of Medicine*, titled "Primary Prevention of Cardiovascular Disease with a Mediterranean Diet" confirmed that among persons at high risk for cardiovascular disease, a Mediterranean diet supplemented with extra-virgin olive oil or nuts reduced the incidence of major cardiovascular events, primarily stroke.

Another publication in the medical journal *Neurology* in April 2013 revealed that higher adherence to this approach to food consumption was associated with a lower likelihood of cognitive impairment (i.e. dementia). Another study published in the *Journal of the American Medical Association* showed that greater physical activity *and* greater adherence to the Mediterranean diet greatly reduced the risk of Alzheimer's disease. Let's face it. **No** medicine can offer all of these benefits.

What does the U.S. government have to say about healthy eating? In January 2011, the U.S. Department of Agriculture and the U.S. Department of Health and Human Services released the *Dietary Guidelines for Americans 2010* with twenty-three key recommendations (www.dietaryguidelines.gov).

While not specifically recommending the Mediterranean diet, the guidelines are quite similar. The food pyramid is gone, replaced with a plate divided into unequal quadrants for fruits, vegetables, grains (preferably whole grains) and protein (lean) with a small circle off to the side for diary (fat free or low fat). Utilizing this approach, over three-fourths of our food should be fruits, veggies, and grains with less than one-fourth meat. The emphasis is on consuming nutrient-dense foods and avoiding calorie-dense foods and beverages low in nutritional value.

The scientific medical data and the U.S. guidelines point us to eating more vegetables, fruits, and whole grains as the majority of our food consumption. I know how difficult it can be to start and maintain a healthy diet. I had to change my food consumption to conform to what the scientific data has confirmed to be healthy. It wasn't easy. Being born and raised on a farm and ranch, my meals were loaded with eggs, bacon, whole milk, red meat, and potatoes—all cooked with lots of butter and lard.

I've since changed my diet. I feel better and it's much easier for me to keep my weight where I want it. I had to re-program my mind to eat healthy. I've dramatically decreased breads, pastries, dairy products, pasta, and red meat and replaced them with a lot of whole grains, veggies, fruits, nuts, and fish.

If you are the typical American, changing your eating habits to conform to what is proven to be best for our health can be challenging. If my husband and I can do it by slowly making changes over a couple of years, you can do it. We feel so great, we're never going back. Unhealthy foods I thought I could never give up are history.

It is a Culture War—a war we need to win, one meal at a time, by critiquing our caloric consumption and Living WELL Aware.

Essential Element #3:

Make Movement Mandatory!

We all need to "Make Movement Mandatory" in our daily lives. This may be a more palatable term than *exercise*. The problem today is that we are not moving. Without realizing it, we have fallen into a sedentary lifestyle because of today's cultural norms. As compared to the "old days," we are not moving and lifting. Born in 1952 and raised the first twenty years of my life on a farm and ranch, I was hoeing cotton, feeding cows, gathering eggs, and helping Mom cook and clean. I also played basketball in middle school and high school. In fact, physical education was required every year in high school. I moved constantly.

But things are different now. Most kids do not play sports, and physical education is not required every year in many high schools. The street games of yesterday have been replaced with video games and social media. Today, before having even graduated from high school, most adolescents are becoming sedentary.

In addition, technological advancements have drastically decreased our need to move and lift. We have machines and devices to wash our clothes, dry our clothes, wash our dishes, open our garage door, mow our lawn with a self-propelled or riding mower, turn the TV on, drive us around the golf course, get us to the 3rd floor of the building, and get us anywhere we want to go, even if the destination is easily within walking distance. We don't have to walk into the grocery store, buy items to cook food and then carry them into the house and prepare dinner—all of which require a lot of movement. We can just pull through the drive up window and get our greasy tacos, hamburgers, or fries. Or we can just have the pizza delivered to our home.

Most of us also have sedentary jobs, including me. I spend most of my day sitting: talking to patients, working at the computer on research projects, lectures, and newsletters, checking e-mails, dictating patient notes, and talking to colleagues on the phone.

Most of the medical meetings I attend are very unhealthy. We sit all day long and get up only to go to the bathroom or consume enormous amounts of unhealthy calories provided at breakfast, breaks, lunch, and dinner (as if we were working all day and needed all those calories). We have employees at our clinic and hospital who sit all day long because they are answering the phone, assisting with patients' appointments, labs, and other needs.

Does this sound similar to your workday? This is biologically not healthy. We were meant to *move*!

You cannot argue with the data. In addition to Critiquing Caloric Consumption, Making Movement Mandatory is a key element to preventing disease and disability. It is estimated that 5.3 million of the 57 million deaths that occurred worldwide in 2008 were caused by physical inactivity.

The benefits of leading a physically active lifestyle are well established and scientifically proven. Studies have documented that people who remain physically active live longer and have fewer disabilities. They also have lower rates of many cancers. Studies have also reported a direct correlation between increased physical activity and less dementia.

What if you already have cancer? Can physical activity be beneficial? Absolutely! In 2012, the American Cancer Society released Nutrition and Physical Activity Guidelines for Cancer Survivors. Extensive research has been conducted with cancer survivors, focusing on how the benefits of physical activity affect quality of life, cancer recurrence, and long-term survival.

In addition to improving cardiovascular fitness, strength, and self-esteem while reducing fatigue, anxiety, and depression, numerous studies have revealed that physically active cancer survivors have a lower risk of cancer recurrence and improved survival compared to those that were inactive.

Most of the studies showing improved survival involved breast, colorectal, prostate and ovarian cancer patients. Are the over twelve million cancer survivors in the U.S.

aware of this important information? They should be, however doctors may be so focused on treating the cancer, they don't take the time to discuss important lifestyle interventions that can be beneficial. Do most women with breast cancer know that they will probably not die of breast cancer? They are more likely to die of cardiovascular disease, which can be greatly reduced with an active lifestyle along with reducing their risk of breast cancer recurrence.

I am convinced that the only reason my mother made it to two months shy of age eighty-eight was that she refused to stop moving. Despite severe degenerative joint disease, she kept walking. Her orthopedic surgeon was shocked when he saw the X-rays of her ankles and knees and found out she was walking without assistance! She knew that if she quit moving, she would lose her mobility along with her independence. While mom eventually got a walker, this was one of the many examples she taught me on Living WELL Aware. Keep moving if at all possible, even if it is uncomfortable or even at times painful.

How much should we move? When I was growing up on the farm, physical activity guidelines were not necessary. Most people were moving and lifting as part of their daily routine.

Today, guidelines are necessary for most people because of our culture of convenience. According to the *U.S. Department of Health and Human Services Physical Activity*

Guidelines for Americans, adults aged 10 to 64 years should engage in at least 150 minutes per week of moderate intensity or 75 minutes per week of vigorous intensity aerobic physical activity, or an equivalent combination. While some is better than none, surpassing the recommended guidelines is likely to provide even more health benefits. In addition, at least two days per week of muscle-strengthening activities involving all the major muscle groups should be performed.

The American Heart Association released recommendations in 2009 as part of the *Performance Measures for Primary Prevention of Cardiovascular Disease in Adults*. To reduce our risk of chronic disease, we should have 30 minutes of moderately intense activity most days of the week but greater benefits can be achieved from more vigorous or longer activity. This means about 150 minutes per week of exercise that increases your heart rate.

But what about prevention of obesity? To prevent weight gain, we need 60 minutes of moderate to vigorous exercise most days of the week. How much exercise is necessary to assist in weight loss? The guidelines state we need 60 to 90 minutes of daily exercise to help with weight loss. Wow—that's a lot! Let's think about it. Is it really?

We used to get movement in our daily lives before everything was automated for us. We were up and down and up and down, walking here and walking there all over the place. We were lifting, pushing, pulling, washing, and hanging our clothes out to dry. Not anymore. Those 90 minutes when we used to get all of our stuff done now has to be put into our schedule as Making Movement Mandatory.

The good news—it does not have to be all at once. We can work it in throughout the day, starting first thing in the morning. But we have to be creative, working it into our own schedule and finding the things we like to do.

What type of movement am I talking about? In pursuing wellness and searching for optimal fitness, I learned a lot and changed my routine. My husband and I were good about going to the gym routinely to lift some weights to get in resistance training to improve our strength, and we would walk or run on the treadmill for a few miles to increase stamina/cardiac endurance. But we were not working on the important components of balance and flexibility.

It is definitely about survival! Strength, stamina, flexibility, and balance are all important. They decrease our odds of falling and hurting ourselves, increase our bone density, and prevent fractures. They also decrease our risk of heart disease, stroke, dementia, and numerous other disorders including some cancers.

While the scope of all the available ways to exercise are too numerous to include in this book, I will point out some things we should all consider doing to decrease disability and premature death as we age. Of course, you need approval from your provider before starting an exercise program.

Components of Making Movement Mandatory

1. Stamina/Endurance

Move the body forward. Unless you have physical limitations, walking is one of the best forms of movement. It's natural and it's something we all need to do to get around. The faster, the better.

What is considered fast walking? It's about three miles in one hour. That is 20 minutes per mile. It is a goal to work toward if approved by your provider.

Faster is even better, but set reasonable goals when beginning a walking program. If you have a joint problem that keeps you from walking, can it be evaluated and corrected or improved with physical therapy, surgery or medication? My mom would not give up walking. It definitely kept her alive. With the assistance of surgery, medication, and eventually steroid injections, she kept moving.

If you cannot walk, how about swimming, cycling or some other form of activity that gets you moving and gets your heart rate up? Find something you like to do! If you like it, it is easier to keep it up.

2. Strength

Maintain the muscles! As we age, it is quite easy for our muscles to atrophy or to get smaller. When that happens, simple things like getting out of a chair, off the toilet seat, and even lifting light items can become difficult, if not impossible. Visit any assisted-living facility or nursing home for evidence of this. Many of the residents are there because they cannot perform what we in medicine refer to as ADLs, Activities of Daily Living. They simply cannot get out of chairs or walk more than a few steps because they have not retained their muscle mass.

Did our healthcare providers emphasize the importance of standing up and sitting down many times each day? This is what the fitness trainers refer to as "squats." By doing repetitive squats every day we can maintain the strength in our legs. By using simple hand weights, we can maintain muscle mass in our arms.

Going to the bathroom without assistance is something I want to be able to do preferably as long as I am alive. We need to maintain our muscle strength as we age.

3. Balance

OK, I was a klutz most of my life. My balance was horrible. Why? Because I did not work on it. Now I do. I started standing on one foot for a few seconds at a time, and over many months, I slowly increased the amount of time. Now I can stand on one foot and lift hand weights at the same time for several minutes. The better our balance, the less chance we have of falling and hurting ourselves.

4. Flexibility

Having joints that are flexible keeps us from pulling muscles and ligaments and seriously straining our back, neck, hips, and other areas of our body. I didn't realize how bad my flexibility was until I got involved in yoga movements. We all have to start somewhere, and my flexibility is slowly improving.

Being able to have maximum rotation of our hips, shoulders, neck and other areas of our body helps us quickly see the world around us and respond faster to unexpected situations without hurting ourselves.

There are excellent resources to help you Make Movement Mandatory and increase your stamina, strength, balance, and flexibility. It does not require an ex-army sergeant for a personal trainer, a killer boot camp, or running a marathon. You don't even have to go to the gym. There are great *free* programs on line!

It's best to start out slowly and get an accountability partner. We need to question the current culture of convenience. Making Movement Mandatory is key to Living WELL Aware!!

Essential Element #4:

Address Adverse Addictions/ Halt Harmful Habits

We all do some things that are not in our best interest. When we do them repetitively, it can be a major problem. *Addiction* is officially defined by the American Society of Addiction Medicine as, "a primary, chronic disease of brain reward, motivation, memory and related circuitry."

If someone is addicted to heroin or even alcohol, they can have significant withdrawal effects if they abruptly discontinue. Most people do not have true adverse addictions, but we all have certain habits that can be unhealthy in some fashion, physically, emotionally, or spiritually. Some things, in my opinion, are just not good for any of us. I know of no health benefits arising from the use of tobacco products or methamphetamines, or viewing pornography, but I have seen plenty of harm.

Most things are harmful in excess, even food and exercise. Alcohol can be beneficial if you drink only one serving per day. More can lead to numerous problems including difficulties controlling weight, relationship discord, liver cirrhosis and cancer, and accidents, to mention a few. If we have an adverse addiction or harmful habit, it needs to be addressed and halted. Not only can it be physically and emotionally unhealthy, it can also be time consuming and expensive.

We may know some of our habits are detrimental to our life. However, we are often not aware of a harmful addiction or habit. We have transformed some harmful habits into cultural norms and think what we are doing is OK because "everybody's doing it." We do not realize we have a habit of unhealthy eating or excess alcohol eating and drinking similarly.

We may not think that we spend too much time on Facebook, Twitter or checking e-mails because everyone else does too. Then we complain because we don't have time to work out or go to the grocery store and buy healthy food items to cook at home. We think it is OK to charge nonessential things to our credit card knowing we cannot pay them off at the end of the month. Doesn't everybody do that?

We all do some things that keep us from being the awesome person we were meant to be. I have overcome some of mine, and I continue to work on many more. Sometimes I knew what I was doing was not healthy. Other times, it was really a lack of knowledge and awareness.

Now that I'm known as the Wellness Queen and health guru at my hospital and in my community, many are shocked to find I used to smoke up to a pack of cigarettes a day. I even smoked in medical school and residency. I knew smoking was not healthy but continued the habit. I remember thinking that life would not be as enjoyable without smoking. It was a part of my life, a habit. My mind convinced my body that I *needed* cigarettes.

When I got pregnant with our first son, I quit smoking. After he was born, I still occasionally smoked a cigarette. I became a closet smoker because none of the doctors I worked with smoked, and I did not want anyone to know I was partaking in the leading cause of death in the U.S. I eventually did get to the point where I would only smoke if I was traveling, and bummed a cigarette from someone a few times a year, thinking that could not be harmful.

Then one day many years ago I had had enough. I told myself, "I am a nonsmoker." I quit that day and have never smoked a cigarette again. I visualized what even one cigarette was doing to my body, how it was filling my lungs with smoke and introducing harmful chemicals throughout my body, increasing my odds of cancer, heart attack, stroke, and worse yet, wrinkles! I changed my thinking. I went from "I need a cigarette" to "The thought of smoking a cigarette makes me want to throw up."

I knew I had passed the test when several years ago I was at a friend's house and the guys were watching a college football game on an outside backyard TV. They were each smoking a cigar and my friend who was a longtime pack-per-day smoker was having one after another during the game. I had absolutely no desire to light up. I felt great!

To this day, even in stressful times, the thought of having a cigarette does not occur. The mind controls the body, and I've changed my mind forever. I am a nonsmoker. You are what you think! It is never too late to quit smoking. My dad quit at the age of 70 when he started getting short of breath and pain in his legs when he walked. He is now 91 years old and able to walk miles.

What about eating? Until a few years ago, I definitely consumed the typical American diet: red meat, dairy products, processed food, fast food, pastries, carbonated drinks, pizza, and Mexican food. My mind told my body that I needed these types of food and once again, life would not be enjoyable without them. I would be depriving myself of deserved rewards. Yes, I actually thought that. Once again, it was my thinking. Just like I knew cigarette smoking was not good for me, when I began seriously pursuing wellness, it became crystal clear that my food consumption needed a makeover. Part of it was lack of knowledge.

Even though I was a doctor, I didn't receive any education in nutrition, and as a gynecologist I was not up on the latest in healthy eating. I ate what everyone else ate. I slowly started decreasing foods from my diet that were known to increase my risk of disease and replaced them with foods scientifically shown to reduce all types of health disorders. I told myself, "I am a healthy eater." Yes, once again, the body does what the mind tells it to do. My mind told my body I did not need ice cream, cream sauces in my soups or on my fish or veggies, donuts, and pastries. I did not have to have meat with every meal. Starches could be greatly reduced. Fruits and nuts became my snacks instead of refined sugary desserts and candies.

This farm girl converted to a Mediterranean-type diet and so did my husband. The results were soon apparent. We felt better, had more energy, and the fat we were accumulating in undesired locations as we aged into our 50s started to disappear.

My husband, who gave up his nightly big bowl of ice cream, started looking better than ever. He has kept up with his healthy eating and, after 33 years of marriage, looks better than when I married him! We feel so good. We both have vowed, "We're never going back." And importantly, we don't feel like we are missing out on anything.

What is it for you? Is it tobacco use, excess alcohol, unhealthy eating, too much involvement in spectator sports rather than actively playing a sport, gambling, or spending money you do not have? Is it pre-occupation with work or hobbies rather than focusing on your spouse? Do you have habits that lead to a sedentary lifestyle like too much social media, Internet surfing, or watching TV programs that have no socially redeeming value? Are you a shopaholic, buying things that rather than making you healthier and happier are causing turmoil in your life?

We all have some behaviors that we should consider stopping and others we should start. We are creatures of habit, and it is our habits that play the primary role in our health and happiness. We need to Address Adverse Addictions/Halt Harmful Habits if we want to get to the next level of Living WELL Aware!

The Importance of Essential Elements #1, #2, #3, #4:

The 7 Health Metrics

Before we go on to Essential Elements 5 - 11, I need to stop and emphasize the importance of 1 - 4: Normal Numbers Now, Critique Caloric Consumption, Make Movement Mandatory, and Address Adverse Addictions/Halt Harmful Habits.

If we pursue and accomplish these four, we will decrease premature death and disability by meeting scientifically proven health metrics.

The American Heart Association (AHA) developed a set of seven ideal health metrics based on:

1. Smoking status
2. Body mass index (BMI)
3. Dietary assessment
4. Physical activity
5. Cholesterol values
6. Fasting blood sugar
7. Blood pressure (BP)

The ideal state for each health metric category was represented by:

1. Not smoking: never smoked or quit greater than 12 months ago
2. Normal weight: BMI between 18.5 and 25
3. Healthy food consumption: high in vegetables, fruits, and fiber-rich whole grains, low in sodium (less than 1500 mg/day) and low in sugar-sweetened beverages
4. Recommended physical activity: more than 150 minutes per week of moderate or vigorous activity
5. Normal cholesterol: serum total cholesterol less than 200 mg/dL
6. Normal BP: systolic BP less than 120 mm Hg and diastolic BP less than 80 mm Hg
7. Normal blood sugar: fasting blood glucose less than 100 or hemoglobin A_{1c} (HbA_{1c}) less than 5.7%

Data from the Centers for Disease Control and Prevention (CDC) on over seven thousand adults revealed that the more ideal health metrics one meets, the less chance of dying from all causes of death.

Compared with participants who met none of the ideal metrics, those meeting five or greater metrics had a reduction of 78 percent in the risk of dying from any cause, and an 88 percent reduction in risk for death from cardiovascular disease. As Darth Vader said in *The Empire Strikes Back*, "Most Impressive."

How many of the seven ideal health metrics do you meet? In the CDC study, only 1.1 percent met all seven. That's right. Only one in a hundred meet all seven health metrics. So, if you do not meet them all, you are definitely not alone. But, the more you meet, the better.

Most adults met two, three, or four ideal health metrics, all of which are associated with a reduction in mortality compared to those with none. Which ones do you meet? Which ones need some work? Pick one, work on it, get it done, and then pick another.

And what about disability? Another study evaluated over two thousand college graduates aged 60 or greater, assessing three lifestyle risk factors for death and disability:

1) Overweight—BMI greater than 25
2) Current smoker
3) Physical inactivity

The two thousand participants were divided into three groups: low risk (none of the above risk factors), medium risk (only one of the three risk factors), and high risk (two to three risk factors). *Physical inactivity* was defined as absence of vigorous physical activity that works up a sweat (jogging, cycling, brisk walking, swimming, and other sports).

The results showed high blood pressure, lung disease, stomach and bowel disorders, arthritis, and diabetes mellitus were higher in the high-risk group compared with the low-risk group. Those in the low-risk group without risk factors (no smoking, met exercise guidelines, ate a healthy diet) had the lowest disability index. They went an average of 8.0 years longer without disability compared to the high-risk group with at least two of the risk factors. Death rates were approximately 50 percent higher for the high-risk group, compared to the low-risk group.

How fast do you walk? Fairly brisk walking was defined as at least three miles per hour. In this study, faster walking pace was associated with a decrease in disability and death.

So there you have it. We have long term follow-up data on individuals into their eighties and nineties confirming that maintenance of defined health metrics can reduce our risk of dying and becoming disabled. These seven health metrics involve Making Movement Mandatory, Critiquing Caloric Consumption, Normal Numbers Now and Addressing Adverse Addiction/Halting Harmful Habits.

Work with your healthcare provider to have normal numbers. Get rid of unhealthy habits like smoking, unhealthy food consumption, and sedentary living. Push away from the table and pick up the pace! By doing so, we will be Living WELL Aware and providing an example for our family, friends, co-workers, and community. We will also have less need to access the healthcare industry—which is a good thing!

Essential Element #5:

Meticulously Manage Money and Minutes

Now that you know the first four Essential Elements (Make Movement Mandatory, Critique Caloric Consumption, Normal Numbers Now, Address Adverse Addictions/Halt Harmful Habits) that can help us meet the seven health metrics proven to delay death and disability, it should be easy to make it happen, right? You just have to commit to:

- putting fitness in the schedule
- eating healthy
- getting your numbers checked and in the normal range
- halting unhealthy habits such as smoking, sedentary lifestyle, unhealthy eating, over-indulgence in alcohol, etc.

Easier said than done! We all have numerous excuses. The first excuse I hear is, "I don't have enough *time*." The second excuse is, "I don't have enough *money*." And they both are just that—*excuses*. "Meticulously Managing Money and Minutes" is so important that I include it as one of the Essential Elements of Health and Happiness.

If you do not succeed in this aspect of your life, it is impossible to accomplish the other elements.

We spend an enormous amount of time and money consumed with two things—superficial appearance and seeking entertainment. Rather than spending a few bucks on a gym membership, some hand weights, attending a Living WELL Aware seminar, cooking healthy food at home, or reading a book or viewing a program on a wellness topic, we spend an enormous amount of money and time on such things as:

- Removing pubic, chest, and other body hair
- Having pedicures, manicures, and massages
- Coloring, styling and doing other things to our hair
- Removing wrinkles and covering our face with makeup
- Piercing and tattooing body parts
- Buying excessive amounts of clothes and jewelry
- Purchasing houses, cars, pets and other items in excess of our income
- Watching hours of TV programs and movies with negative, unhealthy, and often violent messages
- Spending hours each week surfing the Internet and checking Facebook and Twitter

If you are like me, you can identify with a few of the listed items. If you cannot identify with any of them, I would like to meet you! Are any of the above directly harmful? No, not necessarily.

But in excess, they are extremely harmful if we think they are the answer to true health and happiness, and we do not leave enough time and/or money for things that would increase health and happiness. Now we have a serious problem. We buy into society's false persona of what happiness looks like and how happiness acts. This concept has penetrated our world, often completely without our recognition.

In fact, individuals who refuse to buy into these numerous unhealthy and often expensive and time-consuming activities are considered "weirdos." You become an outlier if you Critique Caloric Consumption, Make Movement Mandatory on a daily basis, and don't watch numerous sitcoms on TV. To that I say, "*Congratulations!*" You are Living WELL Aware.

We are bombarded with messages that tell us we should eat this food, have this possession, look this way, and do this activity. The examples never end. For about a year, I passed a billboard on the way to work exemplifying these dangers. Its insidious, harmful message is rampant today, but I guarantee most people didn't see the danger.

It was a billboard of a middle-aged man sitting in a lounge chair with a drink in his hand on a beautiful beach at a resort. The billboard advertised a local bank and the caption at the top read: "We have a loan for that." A loan for a vacation? I was brought up thinking vacations were something for which you saved, and if you had enough money, you took one. If you didn't, you stayed at home and found other ways to have a good time—which we often did.

I saw another bank ad for loans with a tough-looking guy saying, "I'm just like you. I needed a bigger boat." Oh, really. Are you going to enjoy that boat when something unexpected happens, and you can't make the loan payment? Is the bank going to understand? No, they gottcha.

I was about to conduct a Living WELL Aware seminar for a hospital. They were footing most of the costs, so the registration fee for the one-day event was only $45. I recommended to one of my patients that she consider attending. She was significantly obese with multiple associated medical problems requiring numerous medications. I told her that she would benefit from all the information, implementation suggestions, and inspiration of the speakers.

When she saw the registration fee, she replied that she could not afford it. However, this patient did have enough money to have her hair professionally colored and styled. She had exquisitely applied makeup and perfectly manicured and painted hands and toenails. She also stated that she could not afford to take the day off from work but had announced to me at the beginning of the appointment that she had a vacation to Las Vegas planned. In other words, she had significant time and substantial money for superficial appearance and entertainment, but refused to spend even a small fraction of that amount of time and money working to improve her health.

We all must Meticulously Manage Money and Minutes, and if our health is not a priority, we will not have enough of either left to do the things that *will* help us truly enjoy life and be an example for those around us.

The truth? We are all guilty of spending time doing things that do not serve us well. We spend money on items and activities that we truly do not need and actually may be harmful.

Again, this is a Culture War! Our society says we are "entitled" to things for which we don't have the time or the money. This leads to financial problems, which lead to relationship problems, which lead to stress, which lead to more unhealthy decisions and behaviors. It creates an avalanche of problems building one on the other. We are being sold the idea that we can rack up our debt to a point where we'll never be able to pay it off.

We think this is financial health and happiness. *Not!* One of the biggest reasons for marital discord is financial trouble. Who is the biggest culprit? Our U.S. government has accumulated a multi-trillion dollar debt that our children, grandchildren and great-grandchildren will inherit. And we wonder why young adults are unhealthier and unhappier than ever?

Each of us can look at our lives and find ways to better manage our time and money. While some reading this book may be in the bottom tier of income brackets and others may be "filthy rich," we can all look at what we are doing with our money and determine if it serves us individually and as a society to the best benefit.

Thinking of time, we all have 1440 minutes in each day. What are we doing with those minutes? We'll know we are successful in Meticulously Managing Money and Minutes when we have the time and resources to Graciously Give Our Gifts.

Essential Element #6:

Graciously Give Our Gifts

What does *giving* have to do with health? If we study psychology, we learn that there are several emotional human needs to pursue a meaningful life. Again, optimal health and happiness is not just about MMM, CCC, NNN, and AAA/HHH. It is so much more than that. While they are worded and organized in various ways, I prefer to break down these human needs into categories:

- Connection/Love
- Security/Certainty
- Uncertainty/Variety
- Purpose/Significance
- Growth/Contribution

Those that meet these human needs in healthy ways are the happiest people I know. Being loved, feeling secure and safe, having variety in our lives rather than doing the same things over and over, and finding significance and purpose in what we do are all determinants of our well-being.

What about growth and contribution? Eleanor Roosevelt said it best, "When you cease to make a contribution, you die." If we continually work on growing and striving to be the best model we are capable of being, our contributions will soar as we use our talents to help others. Or, as was so humbly stated by Gandhi, "The best way to find yourself is to lose yourself in the service of others."

What do I want in life? I want to passionately pursue a life that continually lifts me and others to a greater state of well-being: physically, emotionally, and spiritually. The more I am concerned about others rather than myself, the more I am at peace with the world and myself. Give and expect nothing in return. You will never be disappointed.

I do not know how anyone can be healthy and happy without this concept as a major focus of life. Some of my greatest sufferings in life have been in giving and expecting something in return. If you give something and don't get anything back, it was a gift. If you get something back, it was a loan. Our rewards should not be expected while we are on this planet, although they usually are.

Deciding what we give and how we give is as individual and meaningful as life itself. If a billionaire gives away 10 percent of his money equaling $100,000,000, is that as meaningful as someone who makes only $20,000 a year and tithes 10 percent or $2,000? Who will be recognized by our society as being the big donor?

We all know that it is the billionaire that will get recognized while the smaller donor truly had to sacrifice. If I give $10,000 to an orphan center in Africa, is that as meaningful as someone who spends a month working at the center exposing themselves to numerous personal health hazards? Does it matter? Who's counting? It only matters to each of us individually and the meaning we attach to it. Am I giving reluctantly—or graciously? Am I giving the bare minimum or as much as I think I can sacrifice? This is not just about dollars. It is about time.

Yes, we must Meticulously Manage Money and Minutes because when it comes to giving, we are talking about our time, talents and treasures (money). Those of us in the medical field might be tempted to say, "I'm a healthcare professional. I give of myself all day long with my talents." To quote Winston Churchill, "We make a living by what we get. We make a life by what we give." I make a lot of money being a doctor. What do I *give* to make this place a better world?

I find myself at times being selfish with my time and money, pursuing personal gratification and security, hoarding money to make sure I can take care of myself when I'm 150 years of age (OK, maybe 100). There is nothing wrong with responsible saving and personal accountability for our needs in life with the goal of not requiring entitlement programs. In fact, that is my goal. I want to be accountable for my personal health and happiness, including my financial health. I would like to be the part of society that does not add to our growing

U.S. deficit, but instead helps draw it down so that future generations will have less of a burden.

If I pursue wellness and disease prevention, then I am not a part of the growing percentage of our GNP being devoured by healthcare costs. One of the best things I can do for my family is take care of myself: physically, emotionally, spiritually, and financially. By doing so, I am not a burden on them, society, or the taxpayers. What an awesome *gift!* It's worth my weight in gold. Literally!

What if within your family, you all vowed to give the gift of personal health—to take ownership of your life, maximizing your health and happiness. That to me is the greatest gift I could receive.

What a novel idea. What if you told your husband, wife, children, parents, boss, whomever, that you were going to give them an expensive gift. They cannot wear it or drive it but it is going to make their life so much easier. The gift: you are going to make changes that will propel your health to make their lives easier, now and in years to come. I would welcome that gift from anyone and everyone I encounter.

The healthier we are in all aspects of our lives (physically, emotionally, spiritually, financially), the healthier our entire society. The more we are personally accountable for our lives and in addition graciously give to help others, the greater the rewards, here and elsewhere.

But if we want to give the gift of health and happiness to others and ourselves, what's it going to take? Here's the kicker. It is what we do not want to hear because it is totally against what we are told day after day. **We have to inconvenience ourselves.**

We are truly giving when we sacrifice our time, talents, and treasures for others rather than for our own personal benefit. When we stop to help a neighbor, visit a relative or friend in a nursing home, visit the imprisoned, volunteer at a pregnancy crisis center—you name it—it is a sacrifice having no monetary reward. We do it because it's the right thing to do.

Deep down we know what that is. When our actions are in line with what our conscience knows is right and just, we are at peace, and depression and anxiety are kept at bay. We are one step closer to being the best we can be.

I am humbled and privileged to be surrounded by so many friends whose actions motivate me to be a more giving human being. Sherri donates countless hours helping homeless families through her work with Family Promise. Roseann organizes Back Pack Buddies for kids who cannot afford them. Jim ministers to prisoners. Mary Jo visits the elderly in the nursing home. Fallon and Jessica donate time as doctors at the community free clinic. Marcia and Jenny established numerous daycare orphanages in Africa. The list goes on and on.

So many use their time and talents, not receiving anything for it. Well, not a monetary reward. They are getting so much more than that. Why do I want to strive to give more, and more, and more? It is actually a very selfish reason. I want to be happier and thus healthier.

What are you giving that inconveniences you? Make the pledge to personal growth and contribution by making true giving a part of living. By Graciously Giving Our Gifts, we are Living WELL Aware.

Essential Element #7:

FORGIVE: Family, Friends, Foes, and Ourselves

What? I am discussing Essential Elements to Health and Happiness—and #7 is *Forgive?* Yes! Have you noticed the abundance of anger throughout the world? Unless you live in a cave with no satellite, cable, Internet, or cell phone coverage, you cannot escape the problems of anger throughout our society. Anger destroys countries, communities, organizations, businesses, families, and individuals. Forgiveness heals.

There are two situations in which anger is most commonly exhibited:

1) Someone does something to you that makes you acutely angry. It happens all the time. You pick the example. Someone: cuts you off in traffic, steals from you, physically hurts you, misses a deadline, or doesn't give you the promotion, job, or raise.

2) Someone thinks about something in a drastically different way than you do. That person has different beliefs about any one of numerous things: religion, morals, work, rights, lifestyle,

family, money, government policies, or life itself. The list goes on and on. You may believe so strongly about something that it is impossible for you to not get angry with anyone who has opposing views.

It is crucial for our well-being to recognize all the multiple sources of our anger. Emotions are a vital aspect of our health. Our body is one big chemical factory. It functions by releasing an array of substances we call neurotransmitters and hormones. Neuro-transmitters travel within the nerves located throughout our body organs. They keep our heart beating, lungs breathing, and muscles moving. Hormones, such as thyroxine from the thyroid gland, insulin from our pancreas, and steroids from our adrenal gland are vital to regulate our metabolism and growth. Without these substances, we cannot survive. Keeping them in balance helps us function optimally.

When we are angry, our entire body is affected through the immediate release of an array of these neurotransmitter chemicals and hormones. It affects our body functions, physically and emotionally. When we become acutely outraged, these substances can create tense muscles, shallow breathing, rapid heart rate, predictable facial expressions and a host of stomach and bowel problems.

Chronic anger can be even worse. It not only affects our emotional state, but also our physical state. You can probably name someone who seems to always complain about something or be angry about one thing or another. Someone hurt them and they can't get over it: an old boss, a relative, a friend, or a co-worker. Two people have radically different beliefs and ardently disagree.

I am one of those people who could get upset in a heartbeat, or less. If someone said something I remotely disagreed with or did something I didn't want them to do, or did not do something I wanted them to do, I got angry. Sound familiar?

I'm happy to say that I have finally gotten to a stage that when I see myself upset at someone, a warning light goes off in my head. "Patsy, stop, don't be so judgmental. *Listen.* Assess the situation. Where is this person coming from? Why do they think this way? You might actually learn something." I try my best to give this person a chance to speak—without interrupting—and to be totally attentive to what they are saying, rather than thinking about my comeback.

This is so difficult for most of us: being mindful of what someone is saying and where that person is coming from. Rather, we are often mindless of what they are trying to tell us because what we have to say is obviously more important.

Even if I disagree with their action or point of view after hearing them out and thoughtfully thinking it through, getting angry will not help the situation. It will only widen the difference of opinions. Or, as someone I greatly respect often says, "Defense is the first act of war."

What about an unexpected, adverse situation? Ask yourself, "Is getting upset going to help this situation?" The answer is invariably *no*. Ask the second question, "Why am I upset?" It could be something quite legitimate such as my purse was stolen, and now I am going to have to cancel credit cards, get a new driver's license, etc.

But once again, remaining upset is not going to help the situation. I find that I am much more at peace if I think about why someone would steal my purse and be grateful I am not in a situation where I think I have to steal. I can also look inward and ask myself, "Have I ever taken anything in my life that didn't belong to me?" I also find that the sooner I forgive that person, the more at peace I become.

My husband, Jeff, provided a wonderful example for our boys and me of the importance of quickly dumping anger. We were on vacation in Rome on the Metro going to St. Peter's Square. Pope John Paul II would make an appearance. Crowds filled the subway as many headed in the same direction at the same time to see the Pope. Jeff and I had been warned of the pick pocketing in Rome and had fortunately taken precautions; we carried limited money and only one credit card. Jeff even put his wallet in his front pocket and was persistently keeping a hand over it. I am sure you know where this story is heading. Yes, despite all his precautions, and immense pride in implementing them, his wallet was taken out of his front jeans pocket without any awareness on his part. The subway doors opened, people got in and out, and the door quickly closed. My husband felt over his pocket again. Nothing was there.

He looked at me and said, "My wallet's gone."

I replied, "You're kidding me, right?"

He immediately recalled a woman right next to him on the subway who got out expeditiously at the stop. He then knew exactly when it had occurred.

What happened next was even more amazing. Our two young sons were pretty blown away by the incident, as was I. Jeff, though, was cool and calm. What was done was done. By not being focused on anger at the woman who took his wallet, he quickly laid out a plan. Mind you, these were the days before every man, woman, and child had a cell phone. He recalled noticing the American Express office near our hotel. He would go there, cancel the credit card, and get a new one issued.

"You guys head to the square and see the Pope." Jeff didn't want all of us missing a once-in-a-lifetime chance to see the Pope. He arranged a meeting place within the square. The end result: he cancelled the card, arranged for new ones to be sent to our hotel the next day, and met up with us in time to hear the Pope deliver a sermon in several languages.

My husband and I now consider the entire event a blessing. We and our boys experienced the value of controlling anger, assessing a situation, and then expeditiously laying out a plan. We discussed the entire event as a family. We were all thankful that Jeff had Meticulously Managed Money and Minutes.

Only a few dollars and one credit card were taken. Because we left early that morning for our planned event, he had enough time to correct a problem and still join us. We were also grateful that no one was physically harmed.

We also discussed the thief. Why was she stealing from others? Was she trying to feed her family? She was obviously quite accomplished at her occupation, performing it with amazing speed and agility. What upbringing and life circumstances led her to a life of crime?

As my husband discussed the event, there were no emotions of anger. In fact, he related that on his way to join us after canceling the credit card, he prayed for her on the subway. Rather than being angry with her, which would have led to nothing good, he felt sorry for her and fortunate for his own life circumstances. Is Jeff always so cool, calm and collected? He will readily admit—"Hell

No!" He, like most of us, can truly lose it almost on a daily basis.

Find a time when you were really proud of yourself for not getting extremely upset over something unexpected and unwanted, maybe a time when you forgave someone. Recall the event in your mind. How did it make you feel? Even if it is a small incident, it matters. If we relive the serenity of that moment, we are more likely to replicate the behavior in the future, possibly even for something a lot worse.

I am continually amazed at the powerful impact of forgiveness. I have seen people forgive someone who raped them. Some of these women go on to help victims of similar circumstances. Rather than let a negative life event ruin their life, they chose to use it for good to assist others.

I was humbled to hear a father speak about the loss of his child because of a medical error by a hospital pharmacist. An overdose of a medication led to cardiovascular collapse and subsequent death of his son. While he was asked to speak at our hospital to discuss the importance of setting up systems to avoid such medical errors, he made it a point to tell the hundreds of people in attendance that he forgave the pharmacist and was grateful for healthcare professionals who day in and day out make decisions with the life of patients on the line.

This father knew that he had to forgive. To not do so would be a tremendous detriment to his own health and happiness. He had to forgive the pharmacist, not only for her piece of mind, but more importantly, for his.

I'm saddened whenever I hear someone say, "I'll never be able to forgive that person." As the Buddha so correctly said, "You will not be punished for your anger. You will be punished by your anger."

One of the best examples of forgiveness I can think of in modern times is Nelson Mandela. After being imprisoned for 26 years during which time he was often horribly treated, he harbored no anger against those who were responsible for his confinement. After his release, he worked with them for peace in South Africa. A quote often attributed to Mandela sums up the personal importance of forgiveness quite well, "Resentment is like drinking a poison and then hoping it will kill your enemies."

For Christians, Jesus Christ gave the ultimate example. As he died on the cross, he said, "Forgive them for they know not what they do." Every religion and even ancient philosophers proclaim the virtue and necessity of forgiveness. Without it, we carry a burden that weighs us down, often leading to anger, irritability, anxiety, and even depression.

Here lies the sad truth. For many, it may be easier to forgive a stranger for something that was horrendous than our own family or friends for something that occurred years ago and no longer matters. Feelings get hurt and forgiveness seems impossible. I even heard a coworker say that she forgave a relative for something he had done, but still wasn't going to speak to him. Well, then she hasn't forgiven him. As a friend of mine said, "God doesn't ask me to forgive you and love you. He commands me to do so!" It is not an option. He's right.

I still get upset about this and that, but I am delighted to say that I have dumped anger in my life and harbor ill will against no one. Why? Because I'm selfish. I cannot get to the next level of health and happiness if I allow anger to be a roadblock. I will not let it get in my way. Forgiveness is a mandatory component to ultimate health and happiness. When I forgive, I am at my strongest. When I am angry, I am at my weakest. Forgiveness takes away anger, fear, guilt, strain, and so much more. It frees our mind to be the best we can be.

Who is the toughest person for me to forgive? *Me!* I, like all of you, am not perfect. I say and do things I wish I had not. "Patsy, why did you get upset about that? Why didn't you handle that differently?"

Well, in reality, I did what I did. Next time I will know better and will do better. I hope that person forgives me. But if not, I forgive myself. Whom do you need to forgive? Who would like to get a call or even an email from you saying, "Hi! How's it going? Haven't been in touch with you in a while and wanted to see how you were doing? Maybe we can get together sometime." You pick the time, format, and words. By harboring anger, you are harming yourself.

Be selfish by dumping the anger, and you will be propelled on your personal path of Living WELL Aware and better able to Passionately Pursue Purpose and Priorities.

Essential Element #8:

Passionately Pursue Purpose and Priorities

We cannot lead a life of optimal health and true happiness without "Passionately Pursuing Purpose and Priorities." You might ask, Who am I? What are my talents? What is my purpose in life? What are my priorities?

Without a healthy concept of why we are here and what we are truly supposed to be doing, we can find ourselves going through each day not satisfied, complaining, even depressed and anxious, because something seems to be missing. We can robotically go through each day, week, month, and year.

Our priorities may be all out of whack because our purpose in life is ill defined. We may be physically healthy, have plenty of money, be in a loving relationship, and yet something just doesn't seem right. Our life is not in alignment with our purpose.

I believe we are all here for a purpose, each with unique characteristics and abilities. I marvel at the work of so many people I know: computer gurus, special education teachers, motivational and spiritual speakers, mission workers, writers, and artists. We not only have to discover our true talents but use them for good. We need to answer the question—Who am I?

Who am I? It's a critical question for which each of us must have a good answer. And the question is "Who am I?" It is not "What am I?" I could correctly say that I am a mother, wife, sister, daughter, physician, speaker, author, researcher, professor, friend, etc. But who is Patricia (Patsy) Sulak? How would I like people to know me, to describe me? Am I using my talents for good? Why was I created? Without a good answer to, "Who am I?" and "What is my purpose in life?" we might find ourselves spending day after day, year after year, decade after decade, prioritizing things in our lives that do not serve us, our family, or society well. We are not Living WELL Aware.

It is easy to buy into society's definition of who we should be and what we should be doing. And that's exactly what society would like us to do—*buy* our way into health and happiness by purchasing what it has to sell (luxury items, herbal remedies and supplements, body ornaments and makeovers) and spend our valuable time pursuing a means to get them.

We cannot be healthy and happy if we do not accurately define our purpose and priorities so we can appropriately manage our money and minutes. Once again, we must define *who* we are and *what* our purpose in life is. Has this been continually emphasized to you in your life? Was it brought up in high school? In college? In grad school? In religious services? When were you given an assignment to answer the question: Who Am I? Is it something you ask yourself today? Do you continually modify your life to match the ever-evolving answer?

Who am I? Who is Patricia Sulak? I was forced to think about this several years ago at a seminar. The two thousand plus people in the audience were given the individual assignment to define, in one sentence, Who Am I? Not what am I, but *who* am I. I pondered the question all day and into the night. What are my talents? When do I feel the best about my life? When am I most at peace with the world?

My current answer to, "Who is Patricia Sulak?" **I'm a loving, energetic force guided by God to lift others.** That is my goal in life: to love, not hate; to be energetic, not sedentary and lifeless; to be guided by a higher power, not society; to help others, not harm them.

By having a definition of who I am and what my purpose in life is, I can then align my priorities. I have to continually focus on loving others and trying to understand where they are coming from and why they do the things they do. I have to constantly assess why I do the things I do! To be energetic, my physical and emotional health has to be a priority. I cannot lift others without each day lifting myself to higher aspirations.

Even if you do not believe in God, somehow we all are guided in a certain direction by a higher power. Who or what is guiding you? I believe and hope you agree it would be a worthy goal for all to endeavor to lead a life that would make this place a better world—to look for ways to help others rather than continually focusing on our own pleasures.

Once we accurately define who we are and what we really should be doing, it can be downright overwhelming, and even scary. For me, I had to look at my life and assess where I was winning and where I was losing. Being a practicing physician, my life is all about helping others, patient after patient, day after day.

But I was not always understanding and loving when they came to see me with complaints and medical problems that were self-induced. I could bring people down rather than lift them up. I also decided that if I truly wanted to help as many people as I could, I needed to change my career focus. I loved obstetrics and gynecology, and still do. I discerned how my gifts made me unique. I had plenty of awesome colleagues who could deliver babies, perform surgery, and do annual pelvic exams and Pap smears. I felt I was being called to do something else. I was getting restless, day after day, doing the same thing; seeing patient after patient, year after year.

But the real frustration stemmed from the fact that I was not making a significant impact on the biggest health problems my patients faced: self-induced diseases leading to depression, disability and death.

With the passing of each year, I saw health problems in my practice skyrocket. Despite the advances in medicine, patients were unhealthier and unhappier than ever. In less than 25 years, I saw the obesity rate in Texas go from less than 15 percent of the population to over 35 percent and many of them were in my practice. Patients were coming back, year after year, putting on more weight, becoming less physically active, complaining of more and more stressors in life, developing significant medical disorders requiring them to take an assortment of medications, and sometimes requiring surgical procedures to correct the resultant damage.

Despite my attempts to discuss the health hazards of their current behaviors and the benefits of nutritious food consumption, physical activity, and stress reduction, there wasn't enough time in a short office visit to make a major impact on most of my patients. I had 20 to 30 minutes with each patient once a year.

For most healthcare professionals like me in primary care, the majority of this time is spent inquiring about any health complaints, performing a physical exam, troubleshooting any identified problems and prescribing indicated treatments along with ordering any necessary lab work and tests. How much time is left to discuss disease prevention and optimal health? A few minutes maybe—once a year! But my patients were being exposed to unhealthy messages many hours every day of the year. My patients were losing the battle, and so was I.

I needed to answer the questions: Who am I? What are my talents? What is my purpose in life?

The answers can be life altering. They were for me. Doing so helped me assess the problems and the possible answers in not only my patients' lives but my own.

Who am I?

- I'm a loving, energetic force guided by God to lift others.
- The problem: In my medical practice, I'm not able to lift patients out of their self-induced diseases during brief clinic visits.

What are my talents?

- I am an award-winning physician, teacher, researcher, and sought after entertaining speaker at state and national meetings with inspiring, informative messages.
- The problem: My patients are not able to hear me speak for hours at a time. Most of my research, teaching, and clinical work have been in treating disease, not promoting wellness.

What is my purpose in life?

- Improve the well-being of others by using my given and acquired talents.

- The solution: Change my focus from diagnosing and treating disease to preventing disease by accumulating scientifically published data. Develop a program of wellness information, implementation, and—importantly—inspiration. Use my gifts as an engaging, motivating speaker and writer to help others.

Those are the answers to my questions. Who are *you?* What are *your* talents? What is *your* purpose in life? Your answers are critical because they determine your priorities and your ultimate satisfaction with life.

If I define myself as a loving, energetic force guided by God to lift others, and if my purpose is to use my talents as a speaker, writer, and physician to help others, then my priorities will need to be in line with those aspirations. My focus will have to be on health, contribution, and spirituality to mention a few.

I realized that if I think of myself as a tired, overworked, stressed-out person who can't wait for the next vacation cruise and ultimately retirement as the answer to my happiness, my priorities would align in that direction.

How do you see yourself and what are your priorities?

Are these your priorities?

- money
- power
- possessions
- food
- entertainment
- security
- appearance
- revenge
- retirement

Or, are these your priorities?

- family/friends
- self-improvement
- spirituality
- accountability
- health
- forgiveness
- contribution
- to be at peace

It is critically important to define our current priorities and assess what changes we need to make to increase our health and happiness. What priorities are not serving us well? What additions would escalate our lives to levels not yet seen?

My husband, once again, provided a wonderful example for our family when he assessed his priorities. As a urologist in a multispecialty clinic, he had taken on the difficult pediatric urology disorders, many of which required complicated surgeries on babies and young children born with abnormalities. He was trained and boarded as a general urologist but was not board certified in the subspecialty of pediatric urology.

He determined one of his priorities was to be the best pediatric urologic surgeon he could be. He knew this would require extra training. Many excuses could have held him back. "I'm 55 years old." "No one will take this old guy into a training program where the average age is thirty." "My boss won't allow me time away from my institution to do the training anyway." "I'll have to leave my home as there are no training programs in the area." "What will my wife think?" "I will have to take a salary cut as I leave my practice."

Jeff decided to do what Tony Robbins refers to in his book *Awaken the Giant Within*. He *awoke* to what he really had to do to accomplish his desired outcome. He had to give up the stories that were not getting him where he knew he needed to be and erase them, one by one. He had to say: "I'm *not* too old." "I won't know if anyone will take me unless I reach out to them with my goals for providing optimal care to the children I treat." "I won't know if my boss will allow me to take time off unless I actually tell him my desires and my plan." "I need to talk to my wife and discuss the implications of my decision on our relationship, now and in the future."

He did exactly what he said. He got the OK from his boss, his wife, and an outside institution that accepted him into their training program. How? By doing what successful people do. He sold them his idea. He gave up the story of, "I don't have the resources." He embraced the story of, "I'm resourceful. I will make it the way it should be." At the age of 56, he moved to Houston and trained in the subspecialty of pediatric urology. At the age of 58, he became board certified in that subspecialty.

How did he do it? He created a greater awareness of his talents, his priorities, and his desire to be the best he could be to help children with their problems. He gave up the excuses and took ownership of his life.

As an essential human need, we all want our life to have purpose and significance. Why am I here? Does my life matter? In other words, am I obtaining significance in healthy ways? If our primary goal is to make millions of dollars so we can lead a life of luxury and retire early with financial security while leading an extravagant life, then all priorities will focus on making it happen, to the detriment of everything else.

If optimal physical, emotional, and spiritual health is our goal, then we will passionately pursue the best Information, Implementation, and Inspiration to make it happen.

We will define our own personal unique talents and use them to help others and ourselves. We will Meticulously Manage our Money and Minutes to participate in activities and programs that promote wellness. We will change course when necessary as we make adjustments based on what is working and what is not.

On the other hand, if our goal is to turn our health and happiness over to our healthcare providers, and let them give us drugs and surgeries to manage our health, then that is what we will get. If you are not aligning your priorities to passionately pursue personal health, you won't invest time and money to pursue the best disease prevention, physical activity guidelines, dietary recommendations, and stress reduction. You will spend your money and minutes on other things and have the same excuse we hear from patients all day long: I don't have enough time. I don't have enough money.

Your healthcare providers primarily diagnose and treat diseases. They cannot give you optimal physical, emotional, and spiritual health. Only you can do that. If you are relying on your provider for optimal health, happiness and longevity, you are barking up the wrong tree. While my doctor can assist me, she cannot give me optimal health and maximum life expectancy. Only I can do that.

And while Making Movement Mandatory, Critiquing Caloric Consumption, Normal Numbers Now, and Addressing Adverse Addictions are important to our health, optimizing health and happiness is so much more than that. Passionately Pursuing Purpose and Priorities is a lifelong journey filled with rewards that no manicure, sports car, vacation or creamy dessert would ever top.

What if we all set the goal to be the very best we were created to be instead of doing just enough to get by? What if we all were devoted to a lifetime of contribution rather than finding the quickest path to be super rich or to an entitlement program that will take care of us?

What if we all wanted to be accountable for doing all we could personally do to get healthier and happier, rather than relying on the healthcare industry for medications and surgeries? What if we all focused on what we could *give* rather than what we could get? What if we all understood the importance of forgiveness as a critical element of well-being?

You are what you think! Who are you? It is the most important question in life. Why? Because it determines what you are going to passionately pursue and prioritize. By searching for the answers to these questions, I was able to prioritize my time, talents, and treasures to develop a unique wellness program to lift attendees out of self-induced problems onto a path of health and happiness. It also led me to be healthier and happier than I have ever been in my life.

If you are passionately pursuing a worthy purpose, then your priorities will make it happen. The result—you won't be dangerously distracted and diverted by a society filled with convenience, complacency, and consumption.

You will also prioritize other essential elements that will propel you on your personal path of Living WELL Aware. What can keep you from Passionately Pursuing Purpose and Priorities? *Stress!* That is why you must Stifle Stress/Sever Suffering!

Patricia J Sulak MD

Essential Element #9:

Stifle Stress/Sever Suffering

STRESS! Do we go a day without feeling stressed about something? How often do we hear or say:

- "I'm stressed out."
- "I have a stressful job."
- "My kids/spouse/parents/boss/(whomever it is for you) is/are stressing me out."
- "I'm a stress eater."
- "The pain in my back/knee/shoulder/head/ (wherever) is so stressful."
- "I can't stop smoking/lose weight/exercise/ (whatever) because I'm stressed."
- "No one understands the stress I'm under because I can't deal with _____."

What is *stress*? *Stress* is formally defined as: mental or emotional strain or tension resulting from adverse or very demanding circumstances. *Adverse? Demanding?* What determines if something is adverse or demanding? Only one thing—perception! It lies in how we perceive the circumstance. What one views as demanding or stressful, another may view as exciting. Stress can be elicited by either physically or emotionally painful events. Our mind has a huge influence on both.

Consider the stress caused by physical pain. We all know people who seem to have a low pain tolerance, who continually talk about their pain. Others seem to have a high pain threshold and ignore discomfort that would be disabling too many. My mom was one of the toughest people I have ever met.

When my dad informed me that she was having increasing difficulty walking long distances, I took her to see an orthopedic surgeon. He ordered X-rays of her ankle that had been repaired years ago after she fractured it while feeding the cows. (Yes, she was out feeding the cows at age seventy!) The surgeon was a bit shocked when he saw the severity of the degenerative changes in the ankle and also in the knees. He asked what assistance she was using to get around. I told him she wasn't using anything at all.

"A motorized scooter?"

"No."

"A wheelchair?"

"No."

"A walker?"

I again replied, "No."

He looked me right in the eyes and said, "Patsy, hear me out. I'm a tough guy. If these were my legs, I wouldn't be walking! How tough *is* your mom?"

"Kirby," I said, "you have no idea."

My mom ignored pain. She had no time for it. Sometimes this was not a good thing. When my dad told me he noticed she was having difficulty picking up small objects such as coins, I sent her to the hand surgeon who diagnosed severe carpal tunnel syndrome to the point of significant muscle injury due to nerve damage. It is important to listen to our body when we perceive physical pain. Our mind must interpret the meaning and significance, and we must decide the appropriate actions that need to be taken. We can use the sensation of physical pain to warn us and guide us. However, it is of paramount importance that we try to not let it control us. Easier said than done.

I have been humbled many times as I encounter friends and patients dealing with physically painful events. Sarah is a lovely petite lady in her seventies with severe debilitating, deforming rheumatoid arthritis. She saw me annually for her routine exam, arriving in her wheelchair. Always with a beautiful smile on her face, she first asked how my family and I were doing before I ever had a chance to ask her how she was doing.

Although every movement she made had to be painful, she never complained. Because of her severe joint

111

disease, it took three of us to get her on the exam table. When I asked how she was doing, she always replied "Just great. I'm so blessed."

Blessed? I wonder if I could have the same attitude if I had a similar illness and life circumstances. Sarah truly lived the message of: Pain is inevitable. Suffering is Optional! She chose not to focus on her pain, but on the beauty of life around her. As an obstetrician, I've also seen women go through difficult labor with no pain meds, focusing on breathing and a focal point rather than their contractions. Not me. When I was in labor, how did I spell relief? E-P-I-D-U-R-A-L!

I wondered if I could deal with physical pain as well as my mom, Sarah, and so many other people I knew. I had an opportunity a couple of years ago to put myself to the test. While participating in a water sport at the lake, I had the misfortune of totally avulsing my proximal hamstrings off the back of my right upper leg, while skiing on a surfboard. In layman's terms—I ripped my hamstring muscles off my pelvic bone under the buttock region on the back of my upper leg. *Ouch!* The pop was so loud everyone on the motorboat heard it. For a few seconds I suffered excruciating pain. But what happened next was amazing.

While still in the water, I quickly assessed the situation. Something bad has happened but: leg still attached, no bloody water, life jacket still on—not going to drown. Assessment: I'm OK.

My friend who owned the boat quickly brought it around to pick me up. My husband, with a horrific look on his face, asked, "What happened? Are you OK?" I replied, "I think I need a ladder to get back into the boat."

Then he knew something was really wrong because I never needed a ladder to get back in the boat. I hobbled up the ladder holding the back of my leg. He asked if I needed to go to the emergency room. I told him that wouldn't do any good. It was Sunday afternoon and the docs would just give me pain meds until I could see an orthopedic surgeon in the morning.

Since my experience with narcotic pain meds from wisdom teeth removal and knee surgery was associated with horrible side effects (nausea, vomiting, itching, etc.), I knew the best thing for me to do was deal with the pain. I decided to focus on others. I said: "Who's up next for skiing?" And we spent the afternoon, as planned, out on the lake with everyone having a good time. More on what happened next, later.

What about terminal pain? Many of us have experienced being around someone who is dying. Carol and Pam come to mind. Carol was a patient of mine who worked in our hospital. I also took care of her daughters and delivered some of her grandchildren. When she was diagnosed with terminal cancer, she was placed on home hospice, surrounded by her lovely daughters. When I visited her and entered her bedroom, she immediately said: "Patsy, you look tired. Have you been working too hard?"

Pam, a friend from my church with terminal cancer, was just as amazing. She had been admitted into our hospital to see if any treatment options were available. I had been on call all night, which she knew from a mutual friend who was there with her. As soon as I was off call, I went to her hospital room. She attentively looked at me and said, "Patsy, are you getting enough sleep? You look tired."

Excuse Me! Pam and Carol are on their deathbeds, and they're concerned about *my* work hours and sleep. Mind you, if I am dying, I don't know if I'll be concerned about the work hours and sleep hygiene of my visitors. But Carol and Pam were able to deal with death by focusing on life—the lives of the loved ones around them.

What about the stress caused by emotional pain? We can all think of numerous unwanted events such as loss of a job or promotion, financial collapse of a business or personal savings, loss of possessions, news of a personal or family illness such as cancer, death of a loved one, children experiencing difficulties, problems with relatives—the list goes on.

One thing is certain. The events of our lives do not control our emotions. It is the meaning we attach to the events. I am continually humbled as I hear stories of my friends, family, and patients and their response to events they would never have wished to happen. Anyone would consider these events adverse and demanding.

I'll never forget my friend's husband who not only lost his job but also his multi-million dollar retirement when the company he worked for went under. Rather than live a life of misery and regret, he took the "misfortune" to start his own company, subsequently making millions. He looked at the situation as an opportunity to do what he had always wanted to do. I had a friend over for dinner recently. He was told he was going to get the job he had applied for and desired. But, as things turned out, it was given to someone else. He was genuinely looking forward to the job and the salary increase to help take care of his wife and four children. When it fell through, he said to me, "Everything happens for a reason." He even helped the person who got the job he wanted. He refused to be bitter about the situation.

Back to the event out at the lake where I tore my hamstrings off my pelvic bone. While I was doing a pretty good job of dealing with the physical pain, the uncertainty of what needed to be done, and how this injury was going to affect my future physical activities was leading to some emotional uneasiness.

Bill, my orthopedic surgeon and friend, saw me the morning after the injury. After examining me, he was pretty sure I had, indeed, avulsed my hamstring muscles off their attachment to my pelvic bone, but he wanted to confirm the extent of the injury with an MRI. He said: "If you did avulse your hamstrings, I recommend that you get it fixed. Otherwise, you won't be able to do a lot of the running and other activities you're used to doing." OK, I'm thinking: broken, fix it. No problem. I had the MRI done that day. When the results came back, my husband and I went back to his office to look at the pictures taken during the study. Bill sat in front of his computer and pulled up the MRI pictures while I stood behind him viewing the results. Yes, I had indeed ripped my hamstrings off their attachment. But, I'm thinking: broken, fix it. No problem.

What Bill said next, I was not prepared to hear. "If I were you, I'd get this fixed. But, no one here has ever done this type surgery before."

With those words, I immediately felt my heart rate increase and my blood pressure go down. I quickly sat down in the chair by me as I began to feel a bit light headed. I replied: "What do you mean, *no one* here has ever done this type operation before?"

I work at a major medical center, a teaching hospital for a large medical school with an awesome orthopedic department. I was thinking: broken, fix it. No problem. Bill explained that in the past, these injuries were not repaired especially in people my age (I was pushing 59 at that time) because the surgery was complicated and involved operating in a risky area by the sciatic nerve and large blood vessels. Also, hamstrings are not essential to getting around. Having them detached just limited certain activities such as running.

In more recent years, orthopedic surgeons across the country were beginning to repair these injuries with great results, getting people back to their physical status and also preventing the chronic leg pain that can occur later when the detached muscles scar around the sciatic nerve. He related they had been waiting for the right person to come in with such an injury so they could do their *first hamstring attachment.*

OK, I'm working on handling stress and being cool under pressure, but being told I had a problem that no one at my hospital had ever surgically tackled caused my neuroendocrine system to affect my entire body in a split second. I nearly fainted! It was an amazing experience, and I'm glad it happened. It gave me a greater awareness of how our emotions can affect our entire body. Immediately getting control of my emotional state was my goal. And I did. Bill told me about Russell, a gifted young orthopedic surgeon at our hospital who did extremely difficult surgeries including removing cancers from the bones and nerves in the same area as my injury.

I met with Russell that day, discussed the surgery, and he performed it that week. After a lengthy rehab, which I followed religiously, I ran a half marathon the next year. By immediately getting control of my emotional state, I was able to assess all possibilities open to me (including the offer to have the surgery done elsewhere at an institution that had done over a 100 such procedures), make a decision, and follow through. It's not what happens to us in our life. It's the meaning we attach to it. When we control our emotional state, we control our life.

For us moms, one of the most difficult things to do is not worry and stress out over our husband and our children, especially after they reach adulthood. I remember saying (and I feel stupid admitting this), "I'll be happy as long as my husband and boys are happy." I actually said that. In other words, I was holding them hostage to my happiness, rather than finding peace and happiness within my own life. If our happiness depends on others, we are in a heap of trouble and misery.

Stress is inevitable. Suffering is optional. In my pursuit of wellness, I have come across this concept multiple times. I agree. We need to Stifle Stress, and we can then Sever Suffering. How do we decrease the stress in our lives? It does not matter if I am reading the works of Greek philosophers, the Buddha, Confucius, C.S. Lewis, or the New Testament—the answer is the same. We suffer when we argue with reality (or many call it arguing with God).

Rules of Reality cause us to suffer if we deal ineffectively with them. I have narrowed them down to four.

Reality Rule #1: Life is unpredictable. Even though we all know this, it doesn't seem to keep us from stressing out over the unexpected. We wake up each morning hoping things will happen as expected only to experience the unexpected. It may be the traffic jam on the way to an appointment, the unwanted mammogram results, the layoffs at work, or the phone call with bad news about a friend.

Solution to Reality Rule #1: Expect the Unexpected. Rather than each morning waking up hoping that everything will go the way you want, expect the unexpected. Ask yourself, "I wonder what is going to happen today, something not on my radar, that I will need to deal with to Stifle Stress and Sever Suffering?" If we expect the unexpected, we can train ourselves to deal with events in a thoughtful fashion with improved outcomes.

Reality Rule #2: Life is Transient. Most of us believe, or say we believe, that there is a better place after death, usually referred to as heaven. Although often described as the ultimate five-star luxury residency—with no demands, deadlines, or discomforts—none of us seem in a hurry to reach that destination. We cannot control death, but the fear of it can control us. Although we know that death is inevitable and happens unexpectedly every day to many, we hope it won't be a family member, a friend, or us. But, one day it will. Knowing this doesn't seem to prepare us for the inevitable.

Our responses to death are as varied as the causes of death. The age at death doesn't seem to matter. My mom died last year nearing 88 years of age. My dad had just turned 90. They had been married 67 years. My dad lamented that he wished they had just a few more years together. He did not know how he was going to go on without her.

Fortunately, I was able to convince him that all mom ever wanted in life was for him to be happy, and she wasn't going to be too pleased in heaven if he did not go on with his life.

Then there is the opposite end of the life spectrum. While covering labor and delivery at my hospital last year, I was humbled by two events that brought me to my knees. I was called quickly to see a patient who was brought in by ambulance in premature labor. We expeditiously assessed her status, determining she was about to deliver and there was nothing we could do at this advanced stage to stop it. Since she had early prenatal care, we also knew that we would have to tell her that the baby was not old enough to survive.

I gave her the news and said, "I'm so sorry. There's nothing we can do to save the baby when he's born."

I will never forget her response. "Doctor, it's OK. God knows what's best for my baby."

We hugged each other. When the baby was born, she held him for quite a while, loving him during the few minutes he lived. I thought I'd never experience anything like this again.

I was wrong. A few months later I was on call. Late at night, I was awakened to officially pronounce a baby dead. The patient was in labor with a baby who was known to have a lethal birth defect preventing the lungs from developing. Death upon delivery was certain. Unexpectedly, the baby girl did not die immediately so her physician went home for much needed rest. I was called several hours after the delivery when the baby took her last breath.

I am ashamed to say that when I was awakened, I was a bit upset because I was meeting the couple for the first time under such unfortunate circumstances. I entered the room to see a beautiful mother sitting in a chair holding her precious daughter. To get at eye level, I got on my knees and all I could say was: "She's beautiful."

The mom smiled and said, "We are so blessed. We thought we would only have a few minutes to get to know her, but we had several hours."

Blessed? Both of these true events show us a vital truth. It is not what happens to us in life—it is the meaning we attach to it.

How have we handled the deaths of our loved ones? How will we handle future deaths? Since I am several decades old, I have known numerous friends and patients who lost their spouse. Their responses are as different as night and day.

One patient who came for her annual visit announced that her husband had died unexpectedly three months ago. They had been married over 35 years. I asked her how she was doing. She smiled and told me she was not going to live in misery but was going to cherish and honor the time they had together. This was the total opposite of some of my patients, who over ten years after the death of their spouses, "still can't get over his being gone."

My husband and I have discussed this on several occasions. We are both of the mindset that when one of us dies, the other will go on. It will not be the end of life for the survivor. It will just be a different life, and it will be what we make it. A wonderful life!

Solution to Reality Rule #2: Life is precious. Cherish each moment. These three women knew the solution, and implemented it.

Reality Rule #3: I'm not in control of most of life's events. While we can decrease adverse and demanding circumstances and manage many aspects of our lives, we are not in control of most daily events. I cannot control the weather or the traffic. I cannot control what people say about me. I cannot control what people do to me. I cannot control many things that happen in my life.

The solution to Reality Rule #3: I can choose how I react to life's events. One of my major goals in life is to get control of how Patsy reacts to events—favorable or unfavorable. No one has stated this better than Victor Frankl, a survivor of Hitler's concentration camps. He said, "The one thing you can't take away from me is the way I choose to respond to what you do to me. The last of one's freedoms is to choose one's attitude in any given circumstance." Victor Frankl's book, *Man's Search for Meaning*, is a must read for anyone who wants to be at peace, no matter how tragic the life event one may be experiencing.

Reality Rule #4: I am not perfect. This may be the last, but certainly not the least Reality Rule. When I say and do things that hurt others, it's usually because I was thinking of myself and not being mindful. I was not focusing on where someone was coming from and why she said or did what she did. Or, I was trying to be helpful, but could have chosen different words or actions. I do things that personally don't serve me well.

The solution to Reality Rule #4: There is room for improvement! I love the saying, "There are no mistakes, only lessons." As is often said, things happen for a reason. For everything I have done that did not serve others and me well, I can learn from the experience and help others and myself. Until recently, I never understood the phrase, "No Regrets." Now I do. Things *do* happen for a reason. We need to find the reason. What are some things you have done that you wish you had not done? How can you use that experience to the betterment of all?

I have plenty of my own experiences. My son was actually surprised when I said I had no regrets that I smoked for years. I have used that experience to understand and help many with addictions. It also humbles me. We all have things we need to give up that are not serving us well. What are yours? I am working on my list.

What about the times I have hurt people? I can use those experiences to improve my own behavior and be more understanding when people do things that hurt others. In fact, now when my husband and I catch ourselves saying something negative about someone, we try to remember to add the phrase " . . . just like me."

What is it that I am doing or not doing that needs to be improved? If you remember to add that phrase "… just like me" when criticizing others, you may find yourself being more understanding. I do.

I am not perfect! That has power. My goal is to not get older each year. My goal is to get *better* each year. In order for that to happen, there are things I need to do:

1) I need to assess what I truly know needs to be improved in my life: physically, emotionally, and spiritually.

2) I need to find out what needs to be improved that I don't know. In other words, what don't I see? I will never know unless I challenge myself to question what I may have been doing or believing for decades that is not serving humanity or me well. Also, I may not know what needs to be improved unless someone tells me. Cherish people who love you enough to tell you how you can improve. They explain how your actions—or lack of actions—do not serve you well. Rather than getting upset, assess what they say, determine if it would improve your health and well-being, and thank them. That's what I refer to as Relishing Rewarding Relationships: relationships that assist you in achieving the next level of health and happiness.

3) Once I know what changes can get me to the next level of health and happiness, am I willing to change? Phrase it anyway you want, but none of us can get better unless we admit something we are doing or believing needs to change. I do not find this painful. I find this exciting! I hope to be ninety years old thinking, "What do I need to change to get me closer to that best model Patsy Sulak can be?"

Can you imagine how much better our lives would be if we Stifle Stress and Sever Suffering by not arguing with the Rules of Reality but rather work on the solutions? It's mind-boggling. How can we make it happen? We have to Pause/Ponder/Plan/Pray if we are going to be Living WELL Aware.

Essential Element #10:

Periodically PAUSE/PONDER/ PLAN/PRAY

Do things seem overwhelming at this point—MMM, CCC, AAA/HHH, NNN, MMMM, PPPP, GGG, F:FFF, SSSS? I hope not, but if they are, fear not. How can we get off the road of harmful habits and onto the road of healthy habits? We have to stop, then block out all the noise in our environments and in our minds. We need to PAUSE/PONDER/PLAN. Many would also add PRAY. For me, it's about RPM. No, not rotations per minute, it's "Reflection, Prayer, and Meditation."

One would think this process would be the easiest thing to do. I really wanted to spend at least 15 minutes a day to be with myself and no one else. I'd forget about all the things I have to get done and get away from all the electronics, noise, family, friends, co-workers, and pets. I should be able to do that.

Wrong! It is the toughest thing on the list for me to do. I get caught up in all the things I think I need to do and find that life itself is passing me by. I am so focused on the future I miss out on the present. For those of you who successfully do find this time for RPM on a daily basis, I applaud you.

So much of our lives are based on habit. We start out most days doing some of the same things. For example, during the week I get up early in the morning, drink my super greens, go to the gym, come home, have a protein shake with fruit, read the newspaper, have a cup of coffee, shower, brush my teeth, get dressed, go to work. I really don't have to think about it.

The problem is that we can be so programmed in what we do that it conditions us to mindlessly go through the day. Unless we stop and look at our lives we cannot reprogram it for improved habits. In order for us to improve our lives, we have to keep what is working and alter/eliminate what is not working. That requires increasing our awareness of where we are and where we want to be.

I am now in the daily habit of taking a few minutes to stop and just be with myself—no noise, no electronics, no distractions. I first start out with simply being grateful. It is so easy for us to fall into the trap of comparing ourselves to others—a set-up for misery. We are who we are. They are who they are. I am where I am right now in life because that is where I am supposed to be. Arguing with that is insanity!

If we embrace the expected and the unexpected, the gains and the losses, the joy and the sadness of our lives, we can find meaning in all events which creates a greater awareness of who we are and what we can do to have a meaningful life. It is Living Well **AWARE**. If we stop daily and think about the events of our lives and how our actions lead to certain outcomes, we can analyze what went well and what did not. What I often discover is that I was not mindful in many of my actions. I was so concerned about what I wanted to accomplish (the future), I was not present to the moment and the needs of others (the present).

Pausing and pondering allows me to daily take the time to be grateful for all of the many wonderful things about my life: my family, friends, co-workers, and neighbors—as well as my work, and health. It also allows me to assess what I have done and what I have failed to do. What went well yesterday and why? What could have gone better and why?

It reminds me to be attentive to the words, actions, and needs of others. Who needs to be lifted up today? How can I help them? Whom do I need to forgive? Whom do I need to thank?

Why do I need to focus on others? Again, it's because I am selfish. We are all connected to each other in so many ways. My health and happiness is affected by so many, just as theirs is affected by my actions. Practicing mindfulness helps us be present to the moment and to the needs of others.

What does it take to Pause/Ponder/Plan/Pray? In today's world where we are continually connected to each other through text messages, phone calls,

Facebook, Linked-In, Twitter, and email, we need to become momentarily *disconnected*. We must remove ourselves from the constant influx of information through 24/7-world news, financial reports, weather forecasts, politics, sports, and entertainment, so we can just stop and be present to ourselves. We have to briefly forget about the future and all the things we have on our to-do list and take time to do nothing but listen. We have to empty our mind of all thoughts and just be present to the moment. Then we will be able to do what we are called to do.

The benefits of taking a few minutes every day to Pause/Ponder/Plan/Pray are enormous. It blows my mind to think what could happen if everyone just took a few minutes each day to get in touch with their physical, emotional, and spiritual state. What if everyone focused on:

- What they can be grateful for, rather than for what they lack?
- What they did well, rather than only where they "failed"?
- How they can improve their life and the lives of others by utilizing never ending lessons as challenges and opportunities rather than sources of stress, anxiety and depression?

As Albert Einstein so accurately stated, "Problems cannot be solved at the same level of awareness that created them." We must get to a higher level of awareness, and we can only do that if we Periodically Pause, Ponder, Plan, and Play.

Why is this so difficult for most to do? It only takes a few minutes. It costs no money. You do not have to travel to the gym or church or elsewhere. You do not have to dress up. It does not require a partner. There are no physical requirements. You do not have to have a particular religious affiliation or any for that matter.

I think that there are several reasons this essential element to maximal health and happiness is difficult to routinely perform. Here are my reasons:

1) **It can be scary.** To remove ourselves from the noise of the world and assess our physical, emotional, and spiritual state means confronting where we are right now and taking ownership of our lives. This is against our current culture where we are programmed to blame our problems on others, rather than looking at what we can do to make changes in our beliefs and actions to improve our lives. I am elated to have progressed to a point in life where I seek out areas of improvement, areas that need to be changed.

I find it scary *not* to assess my current life and evaluate what I have done that is not in my best interest. Whatever that may be for however long I have been doing it, the sooner I change it, the healthier and happier I will be. That isn't scary. That's exciting! That is living with a life of No Regrets. I can take everything that has happened in my life and learn from it to help others and myself.

2) **We do not see the benefits.** A time of quiet is not like some other activities in which you can actually *see* the results. If you exercise regularly, you will observe increased muscle mass. If you reduce calorie intake, you will notice weight loss. With Periodically Pausing, Pondering, Planning, and Praying, it may be harder to *perceive* the outcomes. We may question how stopping a few minutes to remove ourselves from our chaotic, stressed lives to simply get in touch with our inner selves can be beneficial, especially if no one in our circle is doing it.

The truth is, this is what successful people do. They are always asking, "What don't I see?" "What is keeping me from getting what I want in life?" "What needs to be changed?" They are willing to wait patiently. They know the results may not be immediate. They know they have to periodically pause, ponder and plan to be the best at what they do.

It is not only beneficial to Pause/Ponder/Plan/Pray on a daily basis, but taking longer periods throughout the year is helpful to assess where we are, what we need to change, and create a plan to make it happen. For some, this may be a church retreat, wellness weekend, or self-improvement seminar where time is allowed for personal reflection and growth.

My husband and I plan getaways where we can remove ourselves from the house, work, and all other distractions. We literally put our fast paced lives on Pause as we ponder what we are doing well and not so well, and we come up with a Plan to make it better.

Bill Gates, one of the richest people in the world, truly understands the importance of this concept. Twice a year, he removes himself for a week from his usual professional and private life, and secludes himself at a private location to Pause, Ponder, and Plan his future and that of his company, Microsoft.

All extremely successful people know they cannot get to the next level of where they want to be by doing things the same way. They look for change. They embrace change. They Pause, Ponder and Plan. Doing so will lead them to the foundation of Living WELL Aware as they Seek and Secure Support and Invest in Information, Implementation, and Inspiration.

Essential Element #11:

Seek and Secure Support

Now comes the kicker. How do we accomplish Essential Elements of Health and Happiness 1 – 10? How do we get our numbers normal now, critique caloric consumption, make movement mandatory, address adverse addictions/halt harmful habits, manage money and minutes, graciously give, forgive, passionately pursue purpose and priorities, stifle stress/sever suffering, and pause/ponder/plan/pray? We "Seek and Secure Support." We have to, "Invest in Information, Implementation, and Inspiration" in order to help us on our journeys. And a journey is exactly what it is.

The foundation for a life of health and happiness is the continual pursuit to become that amazing person we are capable of being by seeking the very best information, implementation, and inspiration to get us there. None of us will ever be that perfect model we are capable of being, but if our ultimate goal is to get better each year, month, week, and even day, all the essential elements will begin to fall into place to make it happen.

I will make movement mandatory, critique caloric consumption, get my numbers normal now, address adverse addictions, and halt harmful habits only if my goal is to physically be the best I can be. I will meticulously manage money and minutes and stifle stress and sever suffering only if my goal is to be emotionally the best I can be. I will give, forgive, and practice mindfulness only if my goal is to spiritually be the best I can be.

The rock upon which we build our lives can be as solid as granite or as brittle as sandstone depending on our investment in information, implementation, and inspiration.

Invest in Information: We are continually exposed to information that influences what we believe and the decisions we make. We cannot escape it. They are everywhere! On TV, the Internet, Facebook, Twitter, newspapers, magazines, radio, and billboards—you name it. Seems like everyone has an idea or a product they want to sell you.

If my goal is to travel on a road of health and happiness, then I must continually Invest in Information to keep me on this uphill path to glory. I must also avoid the continual stream of harmful messages that try to sell me this idea or product, promising me ultimate satisfaction, entitlement programs, and an easy downhill path if I'll just do what they say and buy what they're selling. We must question everything! If my goal is to invest in information to be the very best I can be, then I will question what I read, what I view, and what I listen to. And I mean *everything!*

This is the most important decision you can make. *Where* are you spending most of your time getting *what* information? This is crucial. It determines how you think and ultimately what you do and who you are. The mind controls everything. Over the past few years, my husband and I have slowly changed how and where we get our information.

People seek out the information that conveys what is important to them in life. If entertainment, possessions, and superficial appearance are their priority, then they might find themselves spending a significant amount of time:

- Viewing the hottest violent or sexual hit movies, dysfunctional family sitcoms, or sarcastic comedy shows
- Reading gossip magazines on the latest movie star's marital failure and fiction novels on the best seller list that deal with sexual perversion and violence or murder
- Surfing the Internet for the latest version of the iPhone, computer, or whatever technological device that seems to change every six months with must-have options
- Or, last but not least, searching out advertisements, glamour magazines or the shopping channel for the latest cars, clothes, nails, jewelry, shoes, makeup, hair design, _____ (You fill in the blank.)

On the other hand, if your priority is to seek true inner health and happiness by getting one step closer to the best you can be physically, emotionally, spiritually, financially, socially, and intellectually, then you might find yourself:

- Viewing educational programs on TV and DVDs that teach healthy eating and cooking, fitness demonstrations, mindfulness and meditation, world history and geography, religious or spiritual views and opinions, and financial security through savings and debt avoidance
- Reading books and magazines on self-improvement, health, and wellness
- Surfing the Internet for the latest fitness or calorie consumption app
- Attending a wellness program, cooking demo, fitness class, religious service
- Searching for an activity-centered vacation with biking, hiking, snorkeling, skiing, dancing, etc.

I desire to seek out healthy messages and avoid, as much as possible, the unhealthy messages that have caused me pain and misery in my life. Why? Once again, it is because I am selfish. I want the best for Patsy Sulak. I want to be as content as possible, living life to its fullest, and carrying as many people along with me as I can. And by *content*, I do not mean lavish, easy, or having stockpiles of worldly possessions. I refer to being at peace with myself, doing the best I can with what I have.

Why am I so passionate about seeking out the best information? Over the last several decades as a practicing physician, I have seen the ravages of discontent, depression, disability, and even death when one's life is not focused on what brings true joy, peace, and prosperity. I have also seen the development of a culture that dangerously distracts us from being our best.

My husband and I have drastically changed what we watch on TV. Why? As we focused on a life of physical, emotional and spiritual health, we quickly realized most programs portrayed the opposite. Many sit-coms were based on dysfunctional families making them appear as the norm. Other programs centered on violent crimes with graphic images.

Oh, yes, and what about the late night comedy shows we once routinely viewed? Viewing programs with the purpose of finding and making fun out of someone's misfortunes or beliefs that differed from the host were not worth our precious time.

As we worked on mindfulness and being present to others, we also stopped watching talk shows where participants really did not care about mindfully listening to the opposing views, but rather constantly interrupted and argued with each other. We were more inclined to view news programs where people with different opinions received equal time to express their thoughts. I may not agree with someone's point of view, but by thoughtfully listening, I can find out why they believe what they do and make attempts to politely enter into an intelligent discussion of the topic. I might actually learn something.

We also began to choose carefully what books we read. It takes hours of my precious time to read a book. Will this book add or subtract to my ultimate health and happiness? Will this book help me help others? Do I want to read a romance novel or work on having romance in my life? Do I need a book to do that? No, I need to make my husband a major focus of my life.

Rather than watching the latest hot movie of the season, we began viewing educational series on all sorts of topics from mindfulness to healthy eating to fitness to spirituality. What are we listening to? Are the podcasts and radio programs helping me or harming me? Are they filled with positive uplifting messages or comedians ridiculing anything they can find that differs from their own egotistical point of view? When you are truly focused on making your #1 priority in life to be the best you can be, you find yourself questioning many messages on TV, radio, music, Internet, billboards, newspapers, and magazines. Seek out the very best information you can find! Invest in Information!

Invest in Implementation: I think I can guess what many of you are saying now. "I know what I should do. I'm sold on the information. But how do I implement all this in my life?" The answer: slowly, one step, one change at a time, with commitment and determination.

Let's take Critiquing Calorie Consumption. If you are sold on what is healthy eating, then how do you implement it in your daily life? You sit down and Invest in Implementation by coming up with a list of things you *will do right now* such as get unhealthy food out of the house, look for healthy cookbooks and classes, bring your healthy lunch to work, eliminate one unhealthy food at a time from your diet such as high fat dairy. You make your own list of things you will do, not what you should do or might do.

How about Making Movement Mandatory? Same thing. You write down things you *will begin immediately* such as walk every day for one mile, two miles, whatever you will do. Come up with a list of things you can even do at work such as stand most of the day while talking on the phone, take the stairs, park farther away. Find a sport you will participate in rather than just viewing sports on TV. Look for any information that you know will improve your life and quickly write down ways you will slowly begin to implement that information into your schedule.

WARNING: Your mind will tell you, "I can't do that." Perhaps you will give it a try, only to not stick with whatever you implemented. That is why it is critical at the onset to not say, "I will try this." You must say, "I will make these changes. *I am going to do this.*" We all have things that we say we cannot do.

As Yoda said in *Star Wars*: "Always with you What Cannot Be Done. Hear you nothing that I say? You must unlearn what you have learned."

To which Luke Skywalker reluctantly replied, "All right, I'll give it a try."

Yoda answered, "No! Try not. Do, or do not. There is no try."

Once we come up with our to-do lists and implement them into our lives, how do we stay motivated to stay on target?

Invest in Inspiration: There are those out there who may just need the information, and they can implement it all on their own. I am not one of them. I continually Invest in Inspiration to stay on track to get to the next level of where I know I can be. I am inspired by people who take up a new sport or hobby in their 80s, who go from being a couch potato to completing a marathon, who have gone from major depression to a life of peace and contentment, who go from bankruptcy to financial success, who lose over 100 pounds by dumping the excuses and taking ownership of their food consumption and physical activity, who give up bad habits such as tobacco and pornography.

What did they all do? They changed their thinking! "Can't" was replaced with "Will." In order to have the *will* power to stay with the implemented change, it helps to have motivation from multiple sources.

Sometimes it comes from someone who has been there and successfully overcome the obstacle you are trying to tackle. Support groups offer great information, implementation, and, yes, inspiration because one can learn and be inspired by those who have successfully dealt with adversity. Alcoholics Anonymous, Smoke Stoppers, Overeaters Anonymous. These and hundreds of other groups, specific to the situation, are full of people who have been and are where you are. Other sources of inspiration may be an aerobics instructor who pushes you harder than you would ever push yourself, or a friend who will keep you on track, or a health or life coach.

When seeking and securing support, remember that there are no new problems! They are just variations on the same themes. When looking for solutions to your unique situation, you will find that the answers have been there for hundreds of years, if not longer. Thousands of books have been written and conferences conducted by influential people who often have no new information. They are successful at packaging and presenting the concepts in a way that we can relate to as individuals. While I may be inspired to implement the ideas of one author or presenter, another person may not be able to relate to that person at all. We must all find people and programs that give us helpful information, and can assist us in implementing the ideas, while inspiring us to achieve our dreams.

But, as I repeatedly say, "Question Everything." My husband and I have applied many concepts learned from reading books, viewing videos, attending medical meetings, and numerous other conferences. We have also reviewed medical literature and other scientific resources, resulting in our completely dismissing, and even discouraging, some practices that were promoted at seminars and in the media. I invite and encourage you to question the concepts I have outlined in this book. Check them out yourself. Apply what you think will get you to the next level of health and happiness.

Folks, again, there are no new problems! You are just not that unique. Thousands, if not millions, have had the same problems that you have. They're all recycled. And, there are no new answers to what we ourselves can do to improve our current situation. We must learn from others: Greek scholars, spiritual leaders, medical professionals, family, friends, neighbors, colleagues. We must Seek and Secure Support and Invest in Information, Implementation, and Inspiration to get to the next level of health and happiness. That is the foundation of Living WELL Aware.

The original question of this book: Should You FIRE Your Doctor? It needs to be answered. Are your healthcare providers (MD, DO, NP, PA) people you can work with to advance your health status? Are THEY

144

Living WELL Aware? Are they physically fit / energetic? Do they eat healthy? If not, can they inform, instruct, and inspire you to do so? Only you can answer that question. But, remember, it's not up to your HCP to give you optimal health. It is up to YOU! The question is not really "Should You FIRE Your Doctor?" The question is: "Who's on Your team?" Living a life of health and happiness is a team effort. We all need to SEEK and SECURE SUPPORT and our healthcare providers are merely one miniscule component of our overall team. Who is on our spiritual team, your social team, your financial team, your occupational team, your fitness team? I want to Relish Rewarding Relationships and Seek and Secure Support from the best in all areas of my life as I Invest in Information, Implementation, and Inspiration to be a loving energetic force guided by God to lift others.

Making Lasting Changes: How to Prevent Failure!

So, which of my Eleven Essential Elements of Health and Happiness do you need to work on? Remember, this is *my* list of things I am continually working on, perfecting, tweaking, all of which have propelled me, my husband and attendees of my Living WELL Aware conferences to live healthier, happier, more productive lives.

By reading this book and/or attending a Living WELL Aware seminar, most will be motivated to make many changes immediately to improve their current state of well-being. I know this from the evaluations and many e-mails, phone calls, and posts I receive. Some stories reveal amazing transformations from a life of disease and discontent to a life of health and happiness. From morbid obesity to an ideal BMI, couch potato to long distance runner, depression to happiness.

The stories are each about individuals who took the Information, Implementation, and Inspiration provided and combined it with two necessary ingredients: a passion for improvement and a willingness to change. We can have the best information on what is proven to get on this path, the best sources of how to implement the information, and the most inspiring stories and people to motivate us; but it will not and cannot lead to lasting changes if we do not have a personal passion for improving our current state *and* a willingness to dump the stories that are not serving our best interest and *change* our thinking.

Information/Implementation/Inspiration + Passion to Improve + Will to Change = TRANSFORMATION

The data is not debatable. Living WELL Aware, as outlined in the Eleven Essential Elements to Health and Happiness, will not only dramatically decrease death and disability but will propel the lives of those around us. Knowing that, how can we set ourselves up for success to make the lasting changes we need to get closer to that best model of ourselves and by doing so prevent failure? I think there are six things we have to do to get on a successful path of reaching our goals: **Focus, Plan, Monitor, Correct, Seek, and Own.**

FOCUS ON IT If health is a major focus in our lives, it will be the stepping-stone to accomplishing the goals we have outlined. If we wake up each day and say, "I'm a healthy person. I will make healthy choices," then we are more likely to see it happen. If we continually remind ourselves throughout the day, "I'm a healthy person. I make healthy choices," then we won't just do what everyone else is mindlessly doing. I am focused on passionately pursuing purpose and priorities. And Health and Happiness are at the top of the list. Why? I know it is the best for me and ultimately everyone around me.

PLAN IT If we have a specific plan, we have greatly increased the odds of accomplishing goals and getting there in record time. If we don't, we have just set ourselves up for failure. Failure to Plan is Planning to Fail! I repeat: *Failure to Plan is Planning to Fail!* No matter what you want to improve in your life, this holds true. If you want to lose 100 pounds or gain 20 pounds, improve physical fitness, increase financial stability to decrease stress, take your unique skills to the next level, whatever—you must have a specific written plan with immediate, daily, massive action that is put in your schedule.

As an example, if you want to lose or gain weight, what is the immediate, massive, daily plan for your specific goal? One of my rules of medicine as I teach medical students and residents is, "More mistakes are made through lack of thoroughness than lack of knowledge." This is also so true when it comes to making major changes in our lives. We need specific goals and a specific plan to make it happen.

MONITOR IT I learned from a successful businessman an important concept that holds true in many areas of my life—what gets measured gets managed. People get into financial problems because they did not monitor their money and balance expenses and income. They unfortunately bought into the cultural convenience of credit which turns out not to be a convenience at all.

Dave Ramsey is the guru in this arena on helping people monitor their way out of the mess. What about the problems of weight management? If you want to lose or gain weight, then you have to weigh yourself weekly to see if the goal you set has been achieved each week.

If you want to improve your physical fitness, then it is tremendously helpful to record *all* your physical activities daily and monitor progress. How long did you walk each day? How many miles did you walk each week? How many minutes did it take you to walk each mile? Are you getting faster over time? Did it take you 25 minutes to walk that mile at first and then over time you were able to walk it in under 20 minutes, maybe even 15? Are you lifting more pounds with more repetitions? People often get discouraged when they plateau in their progress. Having a record of how far you've come can be the encouragement to build yourself up to get over the hump and move onward. Record. Record. Record!

CORRECT IT Unless you are lucky enough to develop perfect goals and matching plans to make them happen, course correction will be necessary. Some things may just need to be tweaked while others need a major overhaul. You may have set goals that were too aggressive. Perhaps you had an injury, or had to deal with an unexpected life event. You may have tried too much too fast and your life is in chaos.

The weight loss plan, fitness program, or trainer that you selected may not be the right one for you. You may find that you can accomplish more in a shorter amount of time or need more time to reasonably get there. Continual course correction is key. Re-evaluate your goals and plans. Reinforce what's working. Assess what is not working and why. There are no mistakes, only lessons. If something is not working, do not beat yourself into misery. Learn from it, correct it, and move forward!

SEEK IT This is Essential Element #11 again, the foundation of our health and happiness: Seek and Secure Support! This is a *key* element of success or failure. I know so many people who are extremely talented but flounder in one or more areas of life because they are not getting the advice and expertise that will help them in the area of their difficulties.

I have learned that whatever endeavor I pursue, I want to find the best information and people to help me get there. My husband and I wanted to be the very best doctors we could be so we shadowed the best docs we could find. We learned all we could from the very best. We wanted to know what they knew and how to implement what they knew. We were also inspired by the outcomes of their actions. I found ways to get on health committees, advisory boards, and educational forums around the country so I would be able to learn from the leaders in my profession.

When we decided to pursue wellness, we did the same. We knew we had to Seek and Secure Support. We were not going to reinvent the wheel. We had to learn from those smarter and wiser than us. We bought books and DVDs, had some sessions with a personal trainer, and attended wellness conferences. I sought out experts in nutrition, fitness, physical therapy, spirituality, psychology, cardiology, neurology, gastroenterology, and other medical specialties.

What do YOU want to accomplish in your life? Who can help you get there? This is not a sign of weakness. That is a sign of smartness. Wisdom is knowing that you do not know it all and finding someone who does! This is another one of my rules of medicine as a medical school professor, "Don't go down alone. Take your friends with you!"

Some physicians are often reluctant to ask for help or advice, thinking their colleagues will not think favorably of them. This can be a determent to the patient and the doctor, if the desired outcome is not achieved. The same is true of improving our health, and those around us. When it comes to Living WELL Aware, we want to bring those around us up with us as we improve the quality of our lives.

Warning: When you start to make changes, those around you may be your biggest roadblocks. If you begin working on the Essential Elements to Health and Happiness, dramatically deviating from habits of coworkers, friends, or family members, they may suggest that you not bother and try to talk you into doing what they are doing. They may even make fun out of you. Misery loves company! Do not go there. It may come to the point where they no longer want to be around you, or you do not want to be around them. Like-minded people hang out together. People who drink excessively like to hang with people who drink. Those who eat unhealthily hang with people who do the same. On the other hand, people who are into healthy habits like to socialize with those who do likewise.

Whom you spend time with is who you become. Is your peer group health focused, optimistic, energetic, motivating, inspiring, challenging, and moving forward? Or are your friends stagnant, whining, draining, going nowhere, or going downhill? You do not have to dump all relationships that differ from your thinking and actions, but you must determine what will keep you on your path of increasing health and happiness.

OWN IT This is probably the most important when it comes to successfully making lasting changes. Take ownership of the problem and the solution. If I am hit by a drunk driver tomorrow and lose both my legs, I am going to have to take ownership of the condition I am in. It does not matter that I did nothing to contribute to my unfortunate predicament. Being forever angry with the drunk driver and feeling sorry for myself is not going to elevate me out of the situation. Taking ownership of my state and working with everyone around me to deal with it will elevate me.

Whether you weigh 300 pounds, are totally out of shape, are emotionally not where you want to be, have just been fired, cannot get the job you want, have an adverse addiction, or have an incurable cancer, take ownership of where you are. What behaviors contributed to your situation? What behaviors can help you improve your status?

Taking ownership of the situation will propel your progress. Excuses will halt it. Benjamin Franklin correctly stated, "He that is good for making excuses is seldom good for anything else." *Own it!*

Your Personal Health: Answering the Important Questions

1. Who is in charge of your health? It should be obvious at this point. You are! It is up to you to find the best healthcare providers to take a thorough medical history, perform a physical exam, and order appropriate tests to uncover disorders and ideal methods of management. Whether a problem is discovered or not, the Eleven Essential Elements to Health and Happiness are paramount to disease prevention and treatment. You must Invest in the best wellness Information, Implementation and Inspiration to *partner with your provider.* Do not rely solely on your healthcare provider to keep you healthy.

While medical and surgical therapies definitely have their place in treating disease, none can replicate the amazing results of implementing the Eleven Essential Elements of Health and Happiness into your life. If you're on medications for cancer or a serious illness or serious abnormalities of your numbers (ex. high blood pressure, high cholesterol, fasting blood sugar), then by all means, *continue on or begin therapy* as recommended by your provider *as you begin implementing the Essential Elements of Health and Happiness.* You will find that if you follow them, you may need smaller doses of certain medications, fewer medications, or possibly none at all depending on your individual health status. Today, relying less on the healthcare industry should be a goal for us all.

Health is more than the absence of disease. Yes, we do need to commit to memory the seven health metrics of the American Heart Association in order to dramatically decrease death and disability. These seven health metrics do not include aspects of emotional and spiritual health. I can be very healthy according to the health metrics only to be miserable because I'm not giving, forgiving, passionately pursuing purpose and priority, pausing/pondering/planning, and seeking/securing support. Being in charge of your health is taking responsibility for your physical, emotional and spiritual health.

Why do I keep emphasizing this? Because too many of my patients and friends have bought into the idea that if they just show up to their healthcare provider appointments and take their medicines, they will be healthy. *Wrong!* I find it ironic that many of my patients return for their annual appointments, often almost to the exact day of the previous year, thinking that seeing me will protect them from disease and they will be "healthy."

I do not discount routine exams. However, the patients themselves can prevent more diseases than an exam and tests will ever find. Today, many diseases, as we have discussed, are self-induced. We have a Drug Epidemic in this country. We also have a Surgery Epidemic, many of which could have been prevented with a healthy lifestyle. What is the answer? We first need to decide: Who is in charge of my health? If we understand that ultimately we are responsible for our health and happiness, then several other questions need to be answered.

2. What level of health do I want? Physically, emotionally, spiritually, financially, socially? Do you want poor health? Do you want average health? Do you want optimal health? If your answer is "average" health, then that is what you will get.

The "average" person today is in one or probably several of these categories: overweight, stressed out, not in ideal relationships, not following exercise or food consumption guidelines, in debt or solely relying on entitlement programs, not routinely pursuing spiritual guidance, will eventually be on several meds to manage health disorders, and will have greater disability, depression, and earlier death than those who pursue optimal health. That may in itself sound depressing, but it shouldn't. I personally found it exciting knowing that implementing the Essential Elements will readily and reliably reap the rewards.

My husband and I made a **commitment** to pursue **optimal health and happiness**. The results were apparent right away. We physically felt and looked better. More importantly, we were at a higher emotional and spiritual level than we had ever experienced. What level of health do you want? If you now say, "Well of course, I want optimal health," then the next question is paramount to success.

3. Why do I want optimal health? It is important to make a list of all the reasons you want optimal health. Without your personal purpose, you will not stick with the essential elements. I have several reasons on my Why List:

- I want to take as few medications as possible to avoid the inconvenience, expense, possible side effects, and complications associated with them.
- I want to minimize the number of surgical procedures to avoid the inconvenience, pain, expense, and complications.
- I want to feel energetic and be physically fit so I can travel with my family and friends, live independently, and help others.
- I want to be less stressed and angry, and at peace with my life circumstances (planned or unplanned; my doing or not my doing; under my control or not under my control)
- I want to be the solution not the mounting source of today's health and economic problems. I want to be the answer not the excuse.
- I want amazing relationships (family, friends, coworkers, neighbors) where we hold each other accountable, welcome constructive critiques, and

build each other up to be the best we can be individually and as a group to make this a better world.

- I want to be an example for my children, nieces, nephews, friends, and all those around me.

What is your Why List? Be specific. Does it include children, grandchildren, your career, or company? I am not going to make any lasting changes in my life if I do not have a big enough *Why*. Just as I have typed my list, you must also. Then post it so you can continually remind yourself of the reasons you want optimal health. What will it take to have optimal health? It will take w-o-r-k!

4. Am I willing to work for it? It is easy to say that I am going to take charge of my health and seek optimal status. It only takes a few minutes to come up with a Why List. Making it happen is a lifelong commitment. Making Movement Mandatory, Critiquing Caloric Consumption, Stifling Stress and Severing Suffering, etc., cannot be found in a pill. Set yourself up for success. And first and foremost to making it happen is focus.

5. Am I willing to change my focus? This is the ultimate question. If I want to make dramatic changes in my life, I have to change my focus. By making optimal health my focus, I was able to successfully quit smoking, change my food consumption, alter my fitness routine, reduce stress, decrease anger, and have an amazing marriage. I am what I focus on.

When it comes to focusing on optimal health, I don't think about what I am Giving Up. When it comes to increasing my health and happiness, I focus on what I'm Getting Rid Of. I did not Give Up high fat dairy creams and sauces, meat lovers' pizza, processed sandwich meat, greasy sausage, and sugary fat laden pastries. I Got Rid of Them! I did not Give Up cigarettes, sitcom TV, and unhealthy movies, magazines and books. I Got Rid of Them! When health is your focus, replace Give Up with Get Rid. What needs to be on your Get Rid List?

In summary, Should You Fire Your Doctor? Not if your healthcare provider is encouraging you in Living WELL Aware, assisting you in proven recommendations to improve your health, and being an example of optimal health. But remember, healthcare providers will only take your health as seriously as you do. If they feel they are talking to the wall, why should they bother?

On the other hand, if you convey to them that you want to do whatever is within your power to decrease premature death and disability and are making concerted efforts to implement essential elements of health and happiness, they are more likely to step up to the plate and go the extra steps to help you get there. Find a healthcare professional who is knowledgeable in scientifically proven wellness Information, Implementation and Inspiration.

Partner with Your Provider and begin Living WELL Aware!